Michael Denneny, General Editor

Stonewall Inn Editions

Buddies by Ethan Mordden
Joseph and the Old Man by Christopher Davis
Blackbird by Larry Duplechan
Gay Priest by Malcolm Boyd
Privates by Gene Horowitz
Taking Care of Mrs. Carroll by Paul Monette
Conversations with My Elders by Boze Hadleigh
Epidemic of Courage by Lon Nungesser
One Last Waltz by Ethan Mordden
Gay Spirit by Mark Thompson
As If After Sex by Joseph Torchia
The Mayor of Castro Street by Randy Shilts
Nocturnes for the King of Naples by Edmund White
Alienated Affections by Seymour Kleinberg
Sunday's Child by Edward Phillips
The God of Ecstasy by Arthur Evans
Valley of the Shadow by Christopher Davis
Love Alone by Paul Monette
The Boys and Their Baby by Larry Wolff
On Being Gay by Brian McNaught
Parisian Lives by Samuel M. Steward
Living the Spirit by Will Roscoe, ed.
Everybody Loves You by Ethan Mordden
Untold Decades by Robert Patrick
Gay and Lesbian Poetry in Our Time by Carl Morse and Joan Larkin, eds.
Reports from the holocaust: the making of an AIDS activist by Larry
    Kramer

Stonewall Inn Mysteries

Death Takes the Stage by Donald Ward
Sherlock Holmes and the Mysterious Friend of Oscar Wilde by Russell A.
    Brown
A Simple Suburban Murder by Mark Richard Zubro

By Larry Kramer

Fiction
Faggots

Plays
Sissies' Scrapbook
The Normal Heart
Just Say No
The Furniture of Home

Screenplays
Women in Love
The Normal Heart

Nonfiction
Reports from the holocaust:
the making of an AIDS activist

Reports from the holocaust:

the making of an AIDS activist

Larry Kramer

St. Martin's Press
New York

Grateful acknowledgment is made for permission to reprint the following.

"Gay 'Power' Here" © 1978 by The New York Times Company. Reprinted by permission.

"The FDA's Callous Response to AIDS" © 1987 by The New York Times Company. Reprinted by permission.

"An Open Letter to Dr. Anthony Fauci" reprinted by the permission of *The Village Voice*.

REPORTS FROM THE HOLOCAUST: THE MAKING OF AN AIDS AC-TIVIST. Copyright © 1981, 1982, 1983, 1984, 1985, 1986, 1987, 1988, 1989, by Larry Kramer.

Afterword to The Paperback Edition © 1989 by Larry Kramer.

Design by Robin Malkin

Library of Congress Cataloging-in-Publication Data
Kramer, Larry.
    Reports from the holocaust.

    1. AIDS (Disease)—Social aspects—United States.
2. Homosexuality. Male—United States. I. Title.
RC607.A26K73 1989   362.1'9697'9200973   88-34921
ISBN 0-312-02634-X
ISBN 0-312-03836-4 (Pbk)

First Edition
10 9 8 7 6 5 4 3 2 1

For Rodger McFarlane

They have spoken against you everywhere,
But weigh this song with the great and their pride;
I made it out of a mouthful of air,
Their children's children shall say they have lied.

—"He Thinks of Those Who Have
Spoken Evil of His Beloved"
by W. B. Yeats

Contents

ix

Acknowledgments

Many people, some unknowingly, conspire to help one become an "activist." Particularly when, as in my case, I never wanted to be one. If the playwright Robert Chesley had not attacked me one day in 1981, long ago when we were young, in the columns of the gay newspaper the *New York Native,* and if I had not at that time been in therapy with the prescient Dr. Norman Levy, who encouraged me to stop kvetching and respond, I often wonder if I should have been so caught up in what at first was only to be a slight and momentary adjunct to my "other" writing. So, ironically, I must first thank Bob Chesley (and, of course, as always, Norman), and it is to him that my friends and foes can give their gratitude; certainly he has mine.

I thank Chuck Ortleb, the editor-in-chief and publisher of the *Native,* for allowing me the many pages of his newspaper my prose has gobbled up, even when our opinions differed, and his two impeccable editors, first Brett Averill and then Patrick Merla. For those gaffes they caught and I refused to budge on, I take full blame.

Michael Denneny has been all that any writer could ask for in an editor. That he suggested this book puts me in his debt for a start, but the energy and enthusiasm he has lavished on an enterprise that is as far from being a remunerative best-seller as can be imagined have been extremely moving to me. His help on the long essay that is Part Two of this book is particularly acknowledged.

Because I'm convinced everything I've ever written always falls on deaf ears, it is to those who have been kind enough to write or call me, or stop me on the street to offer encouraging words for my efforts, that I also owe appreciation. It's helped keep me going, particularly when I've been roundly criticized, as well as got me back after my periodic burnouts when I vowed Never Again.

No one involved in fighting AIDS does so without the constantly insistent, haunting, painful memories of many too many friends who aren't here in body anymore. They, more than anyone or anything else, have provided all the necessary fuel my energy requires.

My dear loving and loved Rodger McFarlane has lived through all of this with me, and has read, critiqued, and contributed no small input into most of these pieces. He is one of the noblest human beings ever to grace this currently crummy world. This world, and this writer, is lucky to have him, and it is with great admiration, respect, and devotion that I dedicate this book to him.

May he, and I, and everyone still with us, remain among the living.

Introduction

F resh from Yale and the army, I started out, at the beginning of 1958, to do something in the theatre—probably become a producer or an actor; I didn't know yet that I could write. The theatre, then as now, offered precious little opportunity, so, by chance, I found myself working for a movie company. The theatre was forgotten as I attempted to focus my energy and ambition on becoming a film producer. I only half-jokingly wagered with my fellow members of Columbia Pictures' "Executive Training Program" (I ran the teletype machine) that I'd produce my first movie by the time I was thirty. (I almost made it; I was an associate producer at thirty and produced my first film on my own when I was thirty-three.)

I knew I was gay, and there were other homosexuals in the film business with me, but, trying not to think too much about it, we all lived double lives. I duly brought a young woman with me for Monday-night executive screenings when I was assistant to Columbia's head of production in London, and later, when I was assistant to the president of United Artists in New York. I was more interested in learning what my professional talents might be and how to get to the next step on the ladder of success.

I certainly wasn't interested in gay politics. Like many others, when Gay Pride marches started down Fifth Avenue at the end of June, I was on Fire Island. Gay politics had an awful image. Loudmouths, the unkempt, the dirty and unwashed, men in leather or dresses, fat women with greasy, slicked-back ducktail hairdos. Another world. Certainly not a world that connected to mine. Nor did I want it to. On Fire Island, we laughed, in those long-ago days of health, when we watched the evening news on Sunday night flash brief seconds of those straggling, pitiful marches.

There are a lot of us who felt like that, then and now. For me, the change was a slow one. First it took coming to terms with being gay in the first place. That wasn't so easy, and it took many years of psychoanalysis and therapy and many fights with and estrangements from my family. But that's another story. Eventually I not only came to terms with being a gay man, but I came to recognize that I love being one, and want to be no other. That's been, and continues to be, a miraculously wonderful coming of age.

Its onset coincided with a coming of age in my career. I'd produced my movie, and also learned I could write. I wanted to make movies that I could identify with personally. This meant, if not actually dealing entirely with homosexuality, at least including it. I soon discovered this was impossible. The movie industry wasn't interested in any of my concerns. And yet, like all writers discovering themselves, I desperately wanted to write about what I thought and felt. There was no other choice but to try another medium. I wrote a play. It was a resounding failure. I panicked. I quickly wrote a "heterosexual" screenplay and tried to reenter Hollywood. Hollywood again rejected me. When I found most of my daylight hours spent jogging around the complete perimeter of the UCLA campus in Westwood in useless attempts to outrun my anxiety attacks, I came home to New York to write a novel. I was writing my second one when what was to become known as AIDS came along.

It's obviously been sad for me to reread these words of mine, written during the years of AIDS. Depression overcomes me as I count the dead who need not have died. James Baldwin went to his grave filled with anger for the blind hatred against his people, but also with compassion for the frailty of individual man. My anger is still with me, but compassion hasn't arrived yet. And I don't think dying will bring it.

I've always slightly bristled when I'm described as an "activist." It's a word I'm uncomfortable with. I think it's usually meant pejoratively. It's used as a categorizer—to set one apart. I don't think I'm doing anything especially different. I'm a writer writing. I guess the tradition of writers being vociferous political animals is more European than American. Here, this territory comes along with being considered radical, bearded, and unwashed—all the things I had myself disliked in the breed before. I confess to the beard, but I think everything I write and say is eminently sensible, not radical at all. And if one is an "activist," does that mean those who aren't sensible are "passivists" or "pacifists?"

I remember years go, when my novel, *Faggots*, came out, not wanting to be labeled a "gay novelist." I'm a novelist, pure and simple, I huffily defended myself, at the same time demeaningly pushing aside the notion that this novel was in any way a "political act." Well, gay writers have come a long way since 1978. I certainly have. I'm proud to be called a gay novelist, and I certainly realize that almost everything I say and do now falls under the heading "political." Hell—at this period in the history of gay men, just staying alive is a political act.

I guess what I'm trying to say is that I didn't start out to write anything I eventually wrote, but I'm mighty glad I was able to do so. Even if I have to be called an "activist." (I've also been accused of being a "moralist"—my accusers not realizing that nothing they could say would please me more.)

And—if I was a writer writing—I didn't know it then, but I was also a gay man learning as I went along, learning much I had to learn and much I didn't want to learn. Everything was uncharted territory for all of us. Events were happening too quickly to bear. Issues were constantly shifting in importance. And becoming hugely complicated. Quickly we had to master these complications, understand new scientific, medical, pharmaceutical vocabularies, and juggle them adeptly so we could defend ourselves against those who tried to use their presumed "greater" knowledge to lord it over us.

And the cast caught up in playing this morbid drama was coming and, all too frequently, going. And we were all making mistakes faster than we were achieving certain modest wins. We all had hope, then, that if we only worked fast enough . . .

The one question I'm asked more than any other is how I can take all the criticism, attacks, denunciations, slurs, and scorn that have been hurled at me over these years. I don't mean to be simplistic when I say that after a while you get used to it. (And most gay people have had many years of practice.) But as I said, through writing, I've been fortunate to learn many valuable lessons. For starters, I discovered that no matter what you say, x number of people are going to agree with you and x number aren't. So you might as well say what you want to say.

So, to reread these writings from my past—such agonizingly long years, but how did they pass so quickly?—has not only been sad but rather educational. I again realized that not only am I grateful to be alive still (there have been a few days here and there when I wasn't so sure) but that I, along with many others, have grown up.

If being an activist has made both of these possible, I guess there's value in it. But—along with all the others—I know the cost has been too great.

■ ■ ■

To give a sense of the historical context, I've appended notes to most of the pieces, detailing the occasion or other relevant facts that led me to write them.

Part One

Gay "Power" Here

Harvey Milk was shot and killed in San Francisco on November 27th by Dan White. Mr. White also shot and killed Mayor George Moscone. Mr. Moscone wasn't homosexual. Harvey Milk was. He was the first openly acknowledged homosexual ever to be elected to the San Francisco Board of Supervisors, in a city with a homosexual population that is large but not so large as New York's.

I am not a crying man but I had tears in my eyes, as well as shivers of pride, while I was in San Francisco that week, all for a man I had never known and only vaguely heard about.

Thirty thousand people gathered outside City Hall, carrying lit candles in memory of Mayor Moscone and Mr. Milk. Five thousand gathered inside and outside of Temple Emanu-El, and six thousand did the same at the Opera House, with Governor Edumund Brown, Jr., in the front row center, for memorial services for Mr. Milk. There Anne Kronenberg, a lesbian and Mr. Milk's administrative assistant, spoke of his constituents, who loved him. "Harvey understood the necessity of us all working together," she said. The Reverend William H. Barcus

---

* The Op-Ed page of *The New York Times*, December 13, 1978.

of the Church of St. Mary the Virgin, who had recently disclosed his own homosexuality to his congregation, expecting
the worst but receiving warm support instead, asked, "If you
were shot down tomorrow, would the people you love know you
as well as you knew Harvey?" Then Dr. David R. Kessler, a
psychiatrist on the staff of the University of California Medical
School and the Langley-Porter Psychiatric Clinic, and president
of the Bay Area Physicians for Human Rights, a group of more
than 250 homosexual doctors and psychiatrists, spoke: "Harvey
asked us all to come out to our families and friends, to the
people we work with and to those we shop from . . . so that we
can shatter the myth, once and for all, that we were freaks,
weirdos, or sickies . . . Harvey Milk fought for us. Now it is our
turn to fight for him." Inside the Opera House, four thousand
people rose as one to shout.

The new Mayor, Dianne Feinstein, had said, outside City
Hall, "The fact of his homosexuality gave Harvey an insight
into the scars which all oppressed people wear. . . . He believed
that no sacrifice was too great a price to pay for the cause of
human rights."

I returned to New York to discover that our City Council,
on November 29th, had again, for the eighth year, rejected
homosexual human rights. Councilwoman Ruth Messinger said
that the homosexual civil rights bill, which the council refused
to release from committee for full council consideration, involved the rights of "an estimated 10 percent of the population;
on this basis there is a homosexual in one of every three families in every state in the country." She said there were an
estimated one million homosexuals in the city.

I am back in New York, missing, very much, the sense of
community I felt in San Francisco. I call several of my friends,
but no one is home. I know that most of my friends are at the
bars or the baths or the discos, tripping out on trivia.

We haven't had an acknowledged homosexual member of
the City Council representing our constituency. But, gruesomely, I wonder if what happened there should happen here,
would Governor High Carey be in the front row? He has
refused even to meet with the New York Political Action Council, a homosexual professional group organized to interview all
candidates on homosexual issues. Would City Councilwoman

Aileen Ryan make a laudatory speech of tribute? On November 29th, she had said that adequate consideration had been given to the legislation, and urged defeat of the motion.

What temple here would open its doors? The gay rights legislation was actively opposed by Jewish organizations.

Would our one million homosexuals march with lit candles? Will we join with San Francisco's 100,000 homosexuals on July 4th, 1979, in the march on Washington that Harvey Milk was planning at his death?

Where *are* our one million homosexuals?

Several months ago, I listened to Lieutenant Governor-elect Mario Cuomo speak to the homosexual Greater Gotham Business Council. He said that until homosexuals organized, until we prepared accurate demographics on our numbers and our purchasing power, we would get nowhere, that political power—and therefore rights—is based on numbers and money.

I heard Percy Sutton say essentially the same thing two years ago at a very sparsely attended anti–Anita Bryant rally. Mr. Sutton said, in effect: You don't know how many of you there are; until you do, you'll get nowhere.

The City Council was right. We are not ready for our rights in New York. We have not earned them. We have not fought for them. California homosexuals mobilized an entire state to defeat the Briggs Amendment, which would have banned the hiring of homosexual teachers in public schools. New York City's one million homosexuals cannot mobilize a city.

Harvey Milk, William, Barcus, Anne Kronenberg, Dr. David Kessler—we have no one like you here.

Whaen my novel, *Faggots*, was published, the Random House publicity department suggested I write a piece for the Op-Ed page of the *Times*. I'd just returned from promoting the book in, among other cities, San Francisco, and my experiences there formed my debut with what I now see was a purely political statement.

I received a number of phone calls and letters, all
saying, more or less, "Who the fuck are you and what
right do you have publicly mouthing off?" Indeed, I was
criticizing an entire community and its leadership that
I hardly knew and that certainly didn't know me.
"Where have you been all these years, while we've been
working our asses off fighting for the gay rights bill?"
was screamed at me by not a few.

I particularly aroused the wrath of some Jewish
members of the gay synagogue Beth Simchat Torah,
who were offended by my criticism of "Jewish organizations"—by which, of course, I meant heterosexual Jewish organizations, and particularly Orthodox and
Hasidic Jewish organizations. When I was invited to
speak at Beth Simchat Torah, I was barely allowed to do
so, so persistent was the heckling. It was an early and,
at the time, very frightening experience. But a valuable
one. I learned that if one is going to speak one's mind,
best be prepared to get as good as you give. This was
a lesson—violent, vocal, vociferous—I was to learn a
thousand times over with the appearance of *Faggots.*

I thought I'd written a satirical novel about the gay
life I and most of my friends were living. I'd meant it
to be funny. I loved Evelyn Waugh. I would use him as
my model and guide. Everybody would laugh and learn.
It never occured to me that *Faggots* would be *controversial.*

I was completely unprepared for its hostile reception
in certain political quarters. I didn't know then (and I
must confess to not knowing now) what the words
"politically correct" or, in relation to *Faggots,* "politically incorrect" meant. But from these very first appearances I was to learn that, whatever they meant, I
wasn't, to gay leaders, the former, and I most certainly
was the latter.

Even though the book was a best-seller, at the time
I was wounded and frightened by the criticism. I found
myself actually shunned by friends. My best friend
stopped speaking to me, even to this day. People would
cross the street to avoid me, or ignore me at parties, to

a fewer number of which I suddenly found myself invited. On a visit to Fire Island Pines, the summer retreat for many from New York's, and the world's, gay population, and the setting of my novel's concluding section, it was made pointedly clear to me that I was no longer welcome.

For the next three years, until the appearance of what was to become known as AIDS, I kept a pretty low profile. I didn't know it then but I was learning—not originally by choice—that necessary lesson for anyone who insists on speaking his mind: how to become a loner.

A Personal Appeal

I t's difficult to write this without sounding alarmist or too emotional or just plain scared.

If I had written this a month ago, I would have used the figure "40." If I had written this last week, I would have needed "80." Today I must tell you that 120 gay men in the United States—most of them here in New York—are suffering from an often lethal form of cancer called Kaposi's sarcoma or from a virulent form of pneumonia that may be associated with it. More than thirty have died.

By the time you read this, the necessary figures may be much higher.

The men who have been stricken don't appear to have done anything that many New York gay men haven't done at one time or another. We're appalled that this is happening to them and terrified that it could happen to us. It's easy to become frightened that one of the many things we've done or taken over the past years may be all that it takes for a cancer to grow from a tiny something-or-other that got in there who knows when from doing who knows what.

* *New York Native*, Issue 19, August 24–September 6, 1981.

In four months, the number has risen to 120 of us stricken and 30 of us dead.

The majority of Kaposi cases are being tended to at New York University Medical Center. The doctor who is most on top of this situation is there, Dr. Alvin Friedman-Kien. He and his associates are passionately determined to help take care of us and to find out what's going on here.

Money is desperately needed, both for their research, which is going on around the clock, and for the treatment and chemotherapy of many of the patients who have no money or medical insurance.

I hope you will write a check and get your friends to write one, too. This is our disease and we must take care of each other and ourselves. In the past we have often been a divided community; I hope we can all get together on this emergency, undivided, cohesively, and with all the numbers we in so many ways possess.

A few friends had died mysteriously. Several others were sick with unrecognized symptoms. An old friend, Dr. Lawrence Mass, was writing in the *Native* of puzzling appearances of rare cancers and pneumonias in the gay community. And then, on July 3rd, 1981, *The New York Times* ran, buried on an inside page, its first (and for a tragically long nineteen months only one of seven) article, "Rare Cancer Seen in 41 Homosexuals."

I don't know why, but I was scared. I'd had many of the sexually transmitted diseases that the article said I shared with these forty-one homosexuals. I called Larry Mass and he suggested I visit Dr. Alvin Friedman-Kien, at New York University Medical Center, who reported the New York cases. I did so.

The genesis of the above appeal is discussed in the following article.

The First Defense

"**R**ead anything by Kramer closely," Robert Chesley has written to your publication recently [Letters, *Native* 22]. "I think you'll find the subtext is always: the wages of gay sin are death."

I am not interested in sin. I am interested in the difficulties people have in loving each other; I am also interested in how we use sex as a weapon, and I think anyone will find that all of my writing, including my film adaptation of *Women in Love*, concerns itself with explorations of these subjects, which have nothing to do with "the wages of gay sin are death."

Since Bob also suggests—among many other things—that I am self-righteously thrilled by the death of my gay friends from Kaposi's sarcoma (even as I appeal for funds to fight it), I think I must respond beyond the above, even though I have been told it's improper for an author to defend his point of view, his artistic endeavors, or his philosophy in any place other than this artistic work itself. Please excuse me if this response encompasses a rather strange-bedfellowed assortment of topics: death, cancer, my writings, particularly my novel, *Faggots*, and

* *New York Native*, Issue 27, December 21, 1981–January 3, 1982.

my own rather low opinion of our New York gay community as a community. And since it was Bob Chesley who lumped all these subjects together, forgive as well a first-person narrative that might otherwise appear self-serving.

■ ■ ■

I do not understand, and never shall, why criticism of ourselves and some of our actions constitutes "gay homophobia." The literary critic Leslie Fiedler has made the point that only when a minority is mature can it respond to self-criticism in art; and its horrified response to its depiction in anything less than the most "positive" terms is an indication of its immaturity.

■ ■ ■

Bob has not been completely honest with either *Native* readers or his political constituency. We had been friends, and I find it curious that his attacks upon me in print commenced with the cessation of this relationship. From the reporter who arrived at my apartment as a "fan," quoting to me his favorite lines from *Faggots,* effusive in his admiration for it, he turned, rather too suddenly I thought, into someone who has been attacking me in print ever since. His list of my malfeasances is endless. He has already trotted out homophobia, anti-eroticism, self-loathing, sex-as-evil, Anita Bryantism, brainwashed-by-psychoanalysis, fascism.

It has not been necessary for him to drag Kaposi's sarcoma into this and, with the unwitting complicity of the *Native,* to put a symbolic but not less effective damper on our fund-raising campaign. This is outright savagery.

■ ■ ■

I initially involved myself with fund-raising for Kaposi's sarcoma for the simple, uncomplicated reason that three of my friends had died from it. (Now there have been five.) Donald Krintzman, the one among these who was my closest friend, was still alive when he, his good friend and former lover Paul Rapoport, Dr. Lawrence Mass, and I joined together to try to collect funds for the research and treatment being conducted at New York University Medical Center by Donald's doctors, Alvin Friedman-Kien and Linda Laubenstein. Anyone who has read Larry Mass's interview with the "unnamed Kaposi victim" in *Native* issue 19 will understand how a friendship with this extraordinary, courageous man could be so inspirational.

I first learned that Donald had KS last July 29th [1981], when I went to New York University Hospital for information and tests myself. We ran into each other in the waiting room of the laboratory. As we waited for our blood to be drawn, we talked about almost anything else, inanities, rather than confront the coincidence that had brought us together in such a location. Each of us was terrified to ask if the worst was true for his friend. Finally he said, in the firm and confronting way that was to be typical of his death, "Yes, I've got Kaposi's sarcoma."

I had just come from Dr. Friedman-Kien's office upstairs. There I'd seen a young man I recognized. Everything in his expression and posture told me what he'd just been told. He sat down next to me in the waiting room and we nodded to each other and I shook my head softly from side to side in what I hoped would pass for sympathy and understanding. "I don't have anyone I can tell," he finally said to me. "I'm afraid to tell my friends, because they won't understand, and I can't tell my boss or I'll lose my job. There isn't anyone I can talk to." This young man, who is still alive, was the first of the many KS victims whom Donald took under his wing and supplied with his own special tonic of honesty and courage.

Dr. Friedman-Kien had asked me, as someone known in the gay community, to organize a solicitation of funds. He cited several patients who had no medical insurance, and he spoke of his own research. He felt something important was happening with KS: a cancer was occurring in a specific and controlled community; perhaps studying this cancer might reveal something about cancers in general. He also felt it was vital to educate the gay community about the cancer's very existence, and its symptomatology.

He also said he thought what was happening was only the tip of the iceberg. He didn't think what was happening would go away. This was very frightening to me, and still is. He said the numbers would continue to increase. This has unfortunately proved to be correct. There were forty KS-related cases (Kaposi's sarcoma, *Pneumocystis* pneumonia, certain lymphomas) on that day we met, and there are more than 180 cases five months later. Clear-headed friends have pointed out to me that this is not so many, in the scheme of things. Perhaps not. But I still have five friends who have died.

On August 11th, our committee of four held a fund-raiser in my apartment. We called all the friends we could think of who had money for charitable contributions or were well known in the gay community and could help get the word around. Hundreds were invited, including every doctor with a gay practice. Eighty men came.

Donald had prepared contribution circulars, and Dr. Friedman-Kien addressed the gathering and answered questions. He said he thought an epidemic was occurring (it was officially declared such in October by the government) [subsequently to be back-dated to June 5th by the Centers for Disease Control], that the causes were unknown, that there were a number of possible "culprits," none of which could be discounted.

We raised $6,635 as a result of this first night.

Two committees were formed to carry forward the endeavors: one to organize a solicitation of Fire Island, chaired by Philip Gefter, and another to plan a benefit dance, chaired by Edmund White. Each committee had over a dozen members. We all felt we were off to a good start.

■ ■ ■

Bob Chesley is very critical of the appeal I then wrote for the *Native*. This is an appeal the wording of which was approved by Dr. Friedman-Kien and Dr. Mass. I wanted it to be stirring and emotional and thought-provoking and scary. I didn't, and don't, think that anything less than scary was, and is, occurring. Neither does anyone else who has had anything to do with KS. Perhaps if Bob Chesley has had nothing to do with this cancer, it's hard for him to believe it exists. It is hard for me to believe that on August 11th Donald Krintzman was alive and energetically passing out his pledges for contributions in my living room and that on November 12th he was dead from *Pneumocystis* pneumonia and I was attending a memorial service for him at Frank Campbell's, filled with hundreds of men stunned and crying for his loss.

The sentence that has caused Bob, and several other *Native* correspondents, so much difficulty, is medically accurate: "It's easy to become frightened that one of the many things we've done or taken over the past years may be all that it takes for a cancer to grow from a tiny something-or-other that got in there who knows when from doing who knows what." But *something* we are doing *is* ticking off the time bomb that is causing the breakdown of immunity in certain bodies, and while it is true that we don't know what it is specifically, isn't it better to be cautious until various suspected causes have been discounted, rather than be reckless? An individual can choose to continue or cease smoking, where the same warnings have been presented, pointed out to us, and questioned by many. But isn't it stupid to rail against the very presentation of these warnings?

■ ■ ■

Over Labor Day weekend we canvassed Fire Island. Philip Gefter had photocopied several thousand copies of Larry Mass's ground-breaking *Native* article, "Cancer in the Gay Community," which, together with two of Donald's contribution circulars, made a six-page brochure. George Wilson saw to it that one brochure was placed in front of every door in both the Pines and the Grove. Enno Poersch, whose lover Nick Rock was one of the first to die, made posters for our tables, which we manned in the harbors of both communities throughout Saturday and Sunday, and where money could be donated and further information and additional brochures obtained. Jack Fitzsimmons provided cash boxes. Of the original committee formed at my apartment several weeks earlier, only a handful came to the island to help. I cite the following who did help us, and apologize if I have inadvertently overlooked someone: Paul Popham, Enno Poersch, Dr. Jeffrey Marmor, Dr. John Raftis, David Margolis, Joey Hernandez, Mark Rosenberg, Bill Touw.

These people manned the tables with Philip Gefter over the two days. Additionally, Paul Popham (who has in one year lost his lover, Jack Nau, to lymphoblastic lymphoma, and a best friend, Rick Willikoff, to KS) and Rick Fialla and I stood at the door of the Ice Palace on Saturday night with cash boxes. From midnight until 8:00 A.M., from thousands of dancers, we collected $126. The Pines Pavilion would not let us solicit on its premises, despite several appeals.

The entire Labor Day weekend in both communities on Fire Island brought us $769.55. Joey Hernandez went out with a cash box the following weekend and collected a further eighty dollars.

However, checks started coming in through the mail. We comforted ourselves that even if contributions were small at the Island, at least we were educating our community about KS, something few had known anything about before.

■ ■ ■

In four months we have raised $11,806.55. Over half of this money came in from our first fund-raiser in my apartment on August 11th. Five people gave $1,000 each and two people gave $500 each, which means that the rest of the entire gay community in the city of New York has contributed to this cause the sum of $5,806.55

■ ■ ■

Ed White's benefit dance committee was unsuccessful in making any sort of reasonable arrangements with our leading discotheque. Its owner's demands were too greedy. (The benefit has now been set for a Tea Dance on Sunday, January 17th, 1982, at the Paradise Garage.) Appeals to famous gay rock and disco stars, who would not be famous were it not for gay dancers, to appear at this benefit have been turned down.

■ ■ ■

Special solicitations were made to two of the richest homosexuals in the world, without success.

■ ■ ■

The mayor's office was completely unresponsive to our request for any kind of help. Herbert Rickman, who is Mayor Koch's liaison with the gay community, said to me on the phone: "This is something we definitely want to get involved with. I'll get back to you tomorrow." We wanted help in getting non-gay press attention for this disease. *The New York Times* had

refused to run special articles prepared and delivered to them
by hand. Even the *Village Voice* has yet to run an article with
any comprehensive information. Rickman has yet to call.

■ ■ ■

I quote now from more of Bob Chesley's letter in the *Native:*

> I think the concealed meaning in Kramer's emotionalism
> is the triumph of guilt: that gay men *deserve* to die for
> their promiscuity. In his novel, *Faggots,* Kramer told us
> that sex is dirty and that we ought not to be doing what
> we're doing. Now, with Kaposi's sarcoma attacking gay
> men, Kramer assumes he knows the cause (maybe it's on
> page 37 of *Faggots?* Or page 237?), and—let's say that it's
> easy to become frightened that Kramer's *real* emotion is
> a sense of having been vindicated, though tragically: he
> told us so, but we didn't listen to him; nooo—we had to
> learn the hard way, and now we're dying.
>   Read anything by Kramer closely. I think you'll find
> that the subtext is always: the wages of gay sin are death.
> I ask you to look closely at Kramer's writing because I
> think it's important for gay people to know whether or not
> they agree with him. I am not downplaying the seriousness
> of Kaposi's sarcoma. But something else is happening
> here, which is also serious: gay homophobia and anti-eroti-
> cism.

In *Faggots,* I set out to try to understand one main issue:
Why did I see so little love between two homosexual men? Love
is what I wanted and want, and what most of the friends I have
say they want, too. Whatever reasons I came up with in my
novel, they, and it, seem to have touched a most responsive
chord in the gay community. The book has sold exceedingly
well and I have received letters from all over the world thank-
ing me for it. Not one of these letters has been negative. I did
not receive one angry or "hate" letter from the entire American
gay community. The only hate letters I have received have been
from the American gay "political" press.
    Can it be, I have begun to wonder, that the gay "political"

press and critics are out of touch with the realities of their audience and their lives? Can it be that these critics are writing for a very small group, quite possibly only each other?

Can it be possible that, as the feminist Vivian Gornick suggests, this reaction from one's own is predictable, that the people with whom one has shared the experience are incapable of seeing their version portrayed in a different way? "No one forgives an interpretation that is at variance with one's own," Gornick has said. "Nobody forgives you for growing up in their presence."

■ ■ ■

Of the sheer floodtide of gay literature which has been appearing over the past three years in America, perhaps nothing has stirred up so much controversy as *Faggots;* perhaps no other title has been so reviled by the gay media; perhaps no title has been so grotesquely misunderstood. . . .

It is one of the macabre ironies of fate that the world's moralists—not to mention gay activists—have branded (and no doubt will continue to brand) *Faggots* as obscene and self-oppressive . . . though they will almost certainly miss the deeper implications of the book. For Larry Kramer . . . has written a deeply moral . . . book.

. . . It is . . . Larry Kramer's sense of . . . unease with the world of instant sex which appears to have annoyed so many of the American activists—those who seem to equate sex with sexual liberation. . . .

—Peter Burton, *Gay News*, London, June 26, 1980

Mr. Kramer's "sin" is that he has accurately put down (in both senses of the expression) the heartless promiscuity of homosexual New York.

Mr. Kramer's view is a personal one—and it must be remembered that anyone's perceptions are distorted through the prism of their beliefs, ideals, desires. . . . Those who read *Faggots* with due care and attention will discover a novel of deep and abiding morality (and morality can never be out of place); bitter, harshly humorous, grotesque, frightening, comic, and as honest as one individual's perceptions can make it.

—Peter Burton, *Gay News*, London, July 10, 1980

Kramer . . . is asking pointed questions about the nature of urban gay lives which most gay men don't want asked . . . the book lays the blame for "our" rotten image at our own doorstep. Kramer accuses his fellow gays of misusing their freedom and shirking their responsibilities to each other as people. "Yes," says Laverne, one of a trio of male characters completed by Patti and Maxine, "we're all out of the closet but we're still in the ghetto and all I see is guys hurting each other and themselves . . . and yes, the world is giving us a bad name and we're giving us a bad name and one of us has to stop and it's not going to be the world."

—Vito Russo, *Gay News*, London, July 10, 1980

The extraordinary moral invective that attends discussion of books . . . in the wake of the Gay Liberation Movement . . . savaged [*Faggots*]. . . . This insistence on optimism in the face of oppression occludes discussion of actual contradictions within our lives, and relegates cultural production to the realm of facile propagandism.

. . . the point is missed both that *Faggots* is a best-seller, an important fact for any Marxist looking at a cultural product, and that *Faggots* might illuminate the material conditions that made it possible and expose the ideological forms through which those conditions are seen.

. . . the move from literary representation of homosexuality . . . to one in which gay men are plural, engaged with each other, creating, choosing, changing partners, are *social*, seems to me to be of emphatic importance. . . . It marks the entry of homosexuality into society, and thereby creates the possibility of deprivatising the experience of homosexuals.

—Philip Derbyshire, *Gay Left 9*, London

What can become of passion when the beloved wallows in the same pleasure-spots, when each dim corner

of the baths reveals him given up to anonymous ca-
resses, when hour after hour his aura fades because the
same carnal evidences cause him to grow pale? This is
the heart of the narrative, the de-mythification of physical love. . . .

Fags [the title in France] . . . dares to dismantle the
mechanism of feelings, it mocks the alibi of "forbidden
sex" in order to underline all the more heavily that the only
question is our identity and, beyond that, the question of
human identity.

. . . We cannot deny that it lays bare the reality of a
universe temporarily without tenderness. This novel has
the merit of shifting its scrutiny, and its analysis from
within is a revolution.

. . . A revolutionary book, *Fags* is one of the rare novels
in which the gay man carves out for himself the hero's
role—entirely for himself. Still a victim? Perhaps, but of
himself, and no longer of the fragile gods whom the
straights have mummified in order to glorify the anguish
of their loins.

—Hugo Marsan, *Le Gai Pied,* Paris, September 1981
(Translated for me by Richard Howard.)

Why has the reception of *Faggots* by the gay press in England
and France been just the reverse of its reception here? Why has
it been possible for my themes and ideas and explorations to be
so well understood overseas and so misunderstood here at
home? What kind of responsible journalism or criticism is represented when a writer like Bob Chesley must use a fatal disease
to attack me and my novel? What kind of repressive community
are we creating for ourselves when a critic can, as George
Whitmore did in *Body Politic,* implore his readers not to buy
or read my book? Or where a bookstore refuses, as the Oscar
Wilde Memorial Bookshop does, to sell my book? I ask in all
reasonableness: What have I written that is so awful that these
almost totalitarian acts can happen? That my novel can still
cause such controversy among our political spokesmen over
three years after its publication is amazing to me and only
supports the theories I've had from the very beginning of these
outcries: I have touched some essential painful truth that some

do not want to look at, and methinks those who protest protest too much.

■ ■ ■

If these political spokesmen are our leaders, where are they leading us? I see no one leading us in an organized plan to gain our civil rights in New York. I see no one making our annual march up Fifth Avenue to Central Park anything other than the messy, straggly, uncoordinated, unconvincing mess it is. Many people claim to speak for us in Central Park; but they are very angry with each other and apparently out of touch with the community that rambles through that park not listening to them.

Unfortunately, all of our political critics haven't learned that it's very easy to criticize and much harder to get anything done.

What does it take for all of us to work together?

■ ■ ■

If KS were a new form of cancer attacking straight people, it would be receiving constant media attention, and pressures from every side would be so great upon the cancer-funding institutions that research would be proceeding with great intensity. The very government agency—the Centers for Disease Control, in Atlanta—that is monitoring KS so slowly is the same CDC that vigorously investigated Legionnaire's disease when it was a national front-page story and Philadelphia was clamoring for results.

Why is Bob Chesley attacking *me?* Why is he not attacking the CDC for taking so long to prepare their epidemiological studies? Why is he not attacking the National Cancer Institute and the American Cancer Society for showing so little interest in KS and forcing Dr. Friedman-Kien to wait months and possibly years for them to fund his research, which has already produced interesting results?

Two new cases of KS are being diagnosed in New York each week. One new case is being diagnosed in the United States *each day.* Nothing is being done by the gay community to insist that the straight community, which controls all the purse strings and attention-getting devices, help us. Why is Bob Chesley not chastising *The New York Times* for ignoring us? Why is he not going after CBS and NBC and ABC for not running any items whatsoever on their programs? A recent new strain of penicillin-resistant gonorrhea among straights made prime-time news headlines for a week.

Why is he not attacking the men on street corners and in sex and head shops who are selling bottles of popper so filled with impurities that a chemical researcher who has analyzed them said they represent "brother killing brother"? Why is he not dunning the pharmaceutical companies to discover less toxic cures more speedily for our most persistent health problem, amebiasis, which has made it almost impossible for us to make love with each other?

Why is he not criticizing our mayor, who is so shabbily two-faced in all his dealings with one of his largest minorities? Are there any gay men or women on the newly formed Mayor's Committee on Minorities? The city's Orientals now have their own local television channel. And why is the mayor not helping us with amebiasis and KS, both of which are public health problems?

And why is Bob Chesley not looking at the "eroticism" that has made gay health such a concern in New York that every gay doctor in this city is, as Dr. Mass puts it, "exhausted"?

Why is Bob Chesley attacking me? Why is he not asking every homosexual in this city: Why are we here? What are we here for?

■ ■ ■

If every homosexual in New York had voted against Edward Koch, he would not be Mayor of New York. How long must it take for this fact to sink in? I beg everyone to think of the power this should entitle us to. Isn't this a far more important issue to deal with than all these petty jealousies and political irrelevancies I read about week after week in our gay press?

And isn't it far more important to try to deal with the fact that more than 180 of us are suffering from potentially lethal cancers and our entire community is doing so little to help them and ourselves?

■ ■ ■

What is this dream world we inhabit? Why is our community
so impotent and lethargic? Is everything *too* good for us? Do
we need Dunkirks before we can organize and fight back? Until
then, can we only hurt each other?

■ ■ ■

I am not glorying in death. I am overwhelmed by it. The death
of my friends. The death of whatever community there is here
in New York. The death of any visible love.

"Whom do we hate most?" George Steiner has asked. And
answered: "We hate most those who ask of us more than we
want to give, who suggest to us that we are far from stretching
to the full height of our own ethical possibility."

I t can be imagined, the barrage of letters that filled the
Native for weeks after this appeared. Happily, the vit-
riol was evenly divided, pro and con. I say "happily" only
because it was good to get *some* public support. I was
also beginning to realize the usefulness of controversy.
It was controversy that helped sell so many copies of
Faggots; it was, and is, controversy that helps an issue
stay before the public, so that more people join in debate, in this process becoming, one hopes, politicized. At
the least, it helps people think about the issues and
perhaps even make up their minds.

In the year between this article and the next, Gay
Men's Health Crisis was officially founded by Nathan
Fain, Dr. Lawrence Mass, Paul Popham, Paul Rapoport,
Edmund White, and me. In a retrospect that, sadly, only
Larry, Edmund, and I are still alive to share, this year
of 1982 and, for me, the year or so following, was an
inspirational time.

Paul Popham—who was a close friend before we had
our painful disagreements on the direction GMHC
should take, disagreements that destroyed a friendship

that was not to be restored until he was on his death-bed—and I supervised the daily running of the organization. For both of us it became a consuming passion—helping, urging, nurturing, watching this small group develop, at first falteringly, but then beginning to grow as increasing numbers of dedicated men and women came to join us. It was one of those rare moments in life when one felt completely utilized, useful, with a true reason to be alive. But this very community zeal, shared by growing numbers who often sought different goals, and who were to be unable to work together politically, was to become, also at first falteringly but then increasingly, an enormous and painful and destructive problem that I don't think has been solved to this day.

Where Are We Now?

Our second *Newsletter* comes to you at a time when the AIDS problem would seem to have reached a very dark day. Medical scientists cannot really tell us much more now than they could six months ago, when our first *Newsletter* came out. The signals we get from responsible medical authorities are confusing, in part because these authorities are confounded by AIDS and very few doctors like to say, "I don't know." Case numbers are doubling every six months. There is an almost 40-percent mortality rate. There are currently three new cases a day nationally and one and a half new cases a day in New York, which still is the city where 50 percent of all cases occur. Gay men still represent 74 percent of all victims. There is the woeful prediction that there will be ten thousand cases in two years' time.

It's very hard for us not to cry out in anger, frustration, fear, desperation, and utter bewilderment, "How many people must die before something happens!"

By "something" we mean a concerted, all-out effort by our community and by our country to make everyone recognize that we are in the midst of the worst epidemic to hit us since

---

* *GMHC Newsletter*, No. 2. Written October 1982, published February 1983.

polio and to mobilize ourselves into the great and effective agency for action and change that this country is capable of becoming in time of emergency.

For it is hard to imagine a worse emergency, or an enemy to match the stealth and horror of this insidious epidemic, an unknown disease that hides itself.

This being so, it seems to us at Gay Men's Health Crisis that there are still too many people who don't know what's going on, or, worse, who act as if they don't know what's going on.

1. The funding for an all-out research assault has been very slow in coming. Our epidemic is already a year and a half old. Although an earlier award provided $2 million to the CDC for AIDS, there is at this moment no money for specific AIDS research pending in either house of Congress.

The National Institutes of Health, which has an annual budget of four billion dollars, has said it will release— "sometime this year"—at least $3 million through their National Cancer Institute and at least $2 million through their National Institute for Allergy and Infectious Diseases. But they have already received $55 million worth of grant requests from hospitals, doctors, scientists, and institutions who have been clamoring to do research into AIDS.

Five million dollars doesn't buy much research these days, or represent much of a commitment on the part of our country, when you consider the number of victims we have sustained, which, as of January 13th [1983], totaled 333 AIDS deaths.

And when we read articles like the following from *The New York Times* of October 10th, 1982, we are angry about the priorities of our country: "The United States Ambassador . . . donated $25 million Friday on behalf of the Reagan Administration to aid relatives of fifty-seven [natives of a small foreign country] killed in a flood and landslide at a mining camp . . . along with a message from President Reagan saying, 'The American people join me in sending sympathy to those injured, their families and the families of those who lost their lives.' "

2. The straight media have been extremely negligent. Remember the almost daily sympathetic attention they lavished on Legionnaire's disease, toxic-shock syndrome, the Tylenol scare, swine flu—victims from all of which total far fewer than we have sustained from AIDS? Now that AIDS is appearing in more heterosexuals, and in babies, the media have recently paid more attention, but, strangely, only a little more.

Constant national media attention helps exert pressure in Washington to release the flow of funds. And without this media attention we have been deprived, for most of the past year and a half, of our nation's main network of communication: how word is spread, information disseminated, alerts sounded. (Six men recognized they had KS lesions from viewing slides that were shown at GMHC's Second Open Forum two months ago.)

Although the *New York Native* has been excellent in keeping its readership constantly apprised of what is happening, the total circulation of all gay publications is unfortunately tiny compared to our total numbers.

So how can we tell each other, *all* of us, that what's happening now is literally a matter of life or death?

3. There has been a great lack of communication between the gay community and the medical/scientific community. Studies are constantly announced and undertaken by people who have only the vaguest notions of how we live. A mere request in the *Native* for volunteers, with a promise of a complete physical examination or some free "test for AIDS," will net more than enough volunteers in a matter of hours. From these men, statistics are garnered, by heterosexuals unsophisticated in our ways, which are then publicized as fact in medical journals and the media. But the men who respond to these requests are most often those at higher risk, and do not necessarily represent a cross-section of the gay community.

4. We want to mention the complex issue of doctors who have felt unable to help guide us through this terrible period. Medical research and health policy must be shaped on local and national levels. It is this policy that will help determine how this epidemic—and our lives—will be han-

dled, as local and federal governments will have no choice but to become involved. The areas of gay health and sexual medicine are still very loosely defined. If we don't field our own experts, representing *us*, fighting for *us*, there is no telling what will happen to us as more and more pressure is brought to bear on officials to "find an answer" and who then might take the path of least resistance and scapegoat gay men.

Thus far, not enough doctors have stepped forward, identified themselves as gay, and pitched in to help on a public level.

5. Here in New York, the meetings GMHC instituted with City Hall have been very slow in achieving results. In no way have we gained the significant acknowledgment of crisis that San Francisco has, with that city's emergency bequest of $300,000 to its AIDS-related endeavors. Indeed, our top-priority request—that our city help us find space that AIDS patients can use for their own lounge and support-group sessions, to be with their own—remains unfulfilled. For lack of permanent space, AIDS and KS support groups have been forced to move around from week to week, often to top-floor walk-ups that KS patients lack the strength to climb.

Working with our city government is a very slow process. We are not discouraged yet, but we are a long way from receiving the recognition gay communities have achieved in such cities as San Francisco, Los Angeles, Houston, and Washington.

6. The gay community itself is not yet united on AIDS. There is one thing we must not allow AIDS to become, and that is a *political* issue among ourselves. It's not. It's a health issue for us. And it's a national public health emergency issue. This may be the hardest task of all for many of us. We've been too accustomed to fear, particularly the fear that our sexual freedom, so hard fought for, will be taken away from us. But we must realize that sex is not the fabric holding our community together; that's a very questionable assumption indeed about our commonality. We must realize that we are much, much more, that we have a sense of self and identity and relating such as exists

in any religion or philosophy or ethnic background, and in
which sex plays no more a role than it does in heterosexual
identity. And if it takes an emergency epidemic to teach us
this lesson, then let this be one of life's ironies.

We all want this epidemic stopped immediately. GMHC is hardly
pleased to report that no miracle drug or cure has shown itself.
And all of us want to know how to live our lives now. All doctors
everywhere dealing with AIDS are under immense stress, and
the most stressed of all are the physicians of New York who
treat large gay populations—a position of truly heartbreaking
frustration. These doctors are telling us to lessen the number of
sexual partners we come in contact with, so that, if a transmissa-
ble agent is the culprit, we will decrease our chances of getting
or giving it. No doctor we know of is trying to make moral
judgments with this advice. Quite the contrary. They cannot
bear to see one more AIDS diagnosis, and so they are understandably in favor of seeing us live at the expense, perhaps, of
our temporarily suspended sexual liberty. But GMHC believes
that each individual must make his own decision.

   Since, as of January 13th, there were 891 cases of AIDS in
thirty-three states, 67 cases in thirteen foreign countries, and
426 cases in New York City, it is hard for us, for the moment,
to refute this advice, though everyone is entitled to decide for
himself.

   All of us, however, must do everything in our power to make
our community and our government and our country recognize
the frightening implications of these rising numbers. We must
orchestrate this concern, locally, nationally, in Washington, and
pray that this country understands that what is happening to
us, and is now happening to heterosexuals, demands immediate
attention. How many of us are carrying within us the seeds of
this mysterious disease? It is hard to live in New York now
without the torment of this question. And how many of us must
die before an effective national plan of attack is begun?

   Listen to these words from Dr. James Curran of the CDC:
"How are we going to spend the next ten years? That's how
long it could take before a causal agent can be found, along
with its cure. We don't have enough people worried about this
yet."

■ ■ ■

Gay Men's Health Crisis is now one year old. We're certainly no longer the bunch of kids who got together and brought you a disco dance. From six men we have grown to more than three hundred men, each of whom is giving a portion of his weekly time to combating AIDS, and we are now a major social service organization without—as yet—any funding from any state, city, or federal sources, only from you, our community.

We have raised over $150,000; given away almost $50,000 to research; printed and distributed some 25,000 copies of our first *Newsletter* (which was so well received that it is used as a training manual in many hospitals and was even requested by the Library of Congress) and at least 100,000 of this one; prepared and distributed 300,000 Health Recommendation Brochures (in English, Spanish, Creole, and French) with a list of symptoms; fielded almost five thousand Hotline emergency calls, which included hundreds of referrals to doctors; created a Patient Service program that includes Crisis Intervention Counselors (who stay with a patient from immediately after diagnosis as having AIDS), individual and group support therapy, a network of buddies to visit and do chores for those who are ill, legal advisers, and financial aid guidance through the complexities of the welfare system; arranged Open Forums for the community to hear and question doctors prominent in AIDS care; arranged contact with representatives of our mayor and congressmen; helped institute measures to protect the community from unsuitably prepared research studies; investigated and registered complaints against improper medical treatment and hospital care; set up training seminars for doctors, psychiatrists, psychologists, social workers, health-care professionals, and concerned laymen in all areas of AIDS concerns, including how to deal with a friend or lover who may be terminally ill; served as a central source for the media so that most of that which has appeared has been accurate and sensitive. And all of the above services have been provided by volunteers and provided free.

That GMHC has accomplished all of this (and mostly in the last six months), and that so many responsible gay men have stepped forward to accomplish all of this, is one of the most inspirational developments ever to occur in the New York gay community. We have never encountered so much love between men as we have felt in GMHC, and watching this organization grow in response to our community's terrible new needs has been one of the most moving experiences we have ever been privileged to share.

We would not be here in such strength without you. You have been responsible as well. That you have continued to send in your checks and volunteer your services or stop a GMHC member in the street and say Thank You—this has been inspirational, too. There are few communities that, when asked, and within the space of one short month, would loan an organization $130,000, interest-free, as 130 men have done, so that we could effectively plan the greatest gay fund-raising event of all time. And, with $60,000 worth of tickets already sold to our Circus before we've even really started our sales campaign, it looks as though you're going to support that as well.

It goes without saying that we desperately need your support to continue. We need your contributions and we need your names for our mailing list and we need you to come to our Circus in Madison Square Garden on April 30. Like every other living, human being, we need you to keep telling us you approve of us and what we're trying to do.

We must not let this awful sense of unknowing that AIDS yet represents divide us. We might all—every one of us—be potential AIDS victims. More than ever before we must fight together now—to help those who are already ill with AIDS, and to help insure our own future on this earth.

—The Board of Gay Men's Health Crisis, Inc.

I t's hard to believe now that there was so much opposition to printing the above lead article on the part of GMHC's Board. The Board, which now numbered eight men (Larry Mass and Nathan Fain, sensing that the fights that were becoming more and more divisive would become even worse, had left the Board to contribute their energy to GMHC as non-Board members), was so terrified to print it that it was circulated, behind my back, and a vote was taken not to run it "as is" unless a number of disclaimers and caveats were included. Since I was the editor of this issue and dealt with the printer myself, I managed to run most of it as I had written it, and got in much hot water for doing so.

Basically, Paul Popham and I differed philosophically on points that were soon to alienate us completely. He was, for a start, a closeted gay man, who was also now president of the board of a gay organization. He felt GMHC should not in any way *tell* people anything, not in any way make up their minds for them. All we could do was pass out the latest word of what was known and said officially about AIDS, which was very little, usually insensitive and homophobic, and quite often spurious.

At great cost to his own health and stamina, Larry Mass, as both a doctor and a writer, was heroic in his never-ceasing efforts to provide accurate medical information regularly in the *Native*. But as the *Native* became known as "the AIDS newspaper," fewer people wanted to read it. Larry, too, would have his fights with the Board to release his impeccable "Medical Answers About AIDS" publications more swiftly and more often.

Paul and the Board were determined not to issue sex recommendations. Or anything that in any way could be construed as moralizing. It must be remembered that this was long before any causative virus had been posited. What if it was discovered that nothing infectious was going around, he asked. We'd look like fools. And we could also have done a lot of damage: the gay community had fought for so long for the sexual freedoms it now enjoyed that any aspersions cast upon the validity of these were bound to be destructive. It had taken so long for gay men to feel good about themselves. Paul's position seemed to be shared by just about everyone else—in and out of GMHC.

I was out to attack every perceived enemy in sight. If the mayor wouldn't meet with us, attack him publicly. If *The New York Times* wouldn't write about AIDS, go after them with pickets. Reagan, doctors, the NIH, the AMA—you name it, I was after it. I'd go on TV and call Koch a pig (I've never been subtle), and be identified with GMHC, and Paul would get very angry at me. (I remember being interviewed by Jane Pauley on "Today" and considering whether I should say Koch was a closeted gay and that was why he was ignoring us, but chickening out and calling him a pig instead.) Because Paul (and several other Board members) were in the closet, and because no one wanted to do it anyway, I did all the media appearances by default. (Not that I didn't want to do so, or wouldn't have fought to do so.) And pretty much everything I'd say, and how I said it, would drive Paul and the Board crazy. Particularly Paul.

He knew he was right and I knew I was right. He was a much better team player than I'll ever be. I'd been a film producer. I thought I was producing GMHC. He'd been an army officer. Both of us were accustomed to getting results and, in very different fashions, having our own way.

Paul, and the Board, which was composed of many of our mutual friends, felt that softer tactics were required. "You get more with honey than with vinegar" was a modus operandi that was urged upon me regularly.

For the first year or so, there was plenty else for Paul and me to do without having to face up to resolving our differences. Many more of our friends were becoming sick and dying. We were also creating an organization that must look after *them*.

1,112 and Counting

If this article doesn't scare the shit out of you, we're in real trouble. If this article doesn't rouse you to anger, fury, rage, and action, gay men may have no future on this earth. Our continued existence depends on just how angry you can get.

I am writing this as Larry Kramer, and I am speaking for myself, and my views are not to be attributed to Gay Men's Health Crisis.

I repeat: Our continued existence as gay men upon the face of this earth is at stake. Unless we fight for our lives, we shall die. In all the history of homosexuality we have never before been so close to death and extinction. Many of us are dying or already dead.

Before I tell you what we must do, let me tell you what is happening to us.

There are now 1,112 cases of serious Acquired Immune Deficiency Syndrome. When we first became worried, there were only 41. In only twenty-eight days, from January 13th to February 9th [1983], there were 164 new cases—and 73 more dead. The total death tally is now 418. Twenty percent of all

---

* *New York Native*, Issue 59, March 14–27, 1983.

cases were registered this January alone. There have been 195 dead in New York City from among 526 victims. Of all serious AIDS cases, 47.3 percent are in the New York metropolitan area.

These are the serious cases of AIDS, which means Kaposi's sarcoma, *Pneumocystis carinii* pneumonia, and other deadly infections. These numbers do not include the thousands of us walking around with what is also being called AIDS: various forms of swollen lymph glands and fatigues that doctors don't know what to label or what they might portend.

The rise in these numbers is terrifying. Whatever is spreading is now spreading faster as more and more people come down with AIDS.

And, for the first time in this epidemic, leading doctors and researchers are finally admitting they don't know what's going on. I find this terrifying too—as terrifying as the alarming rise in numbers. For the first time, doctors are saying out loud and up front, "I don't know."

For two years they weren't talking like this. For two years we've heard a different theory every few weeks. We grasped at the straws of possible cause: promiscuity, poppers, back rooms, the baths, rimming, fisting, anal intercourse, urine, semen, shit, saliva, sweat, blood, blacks, a single virus, a new virus, repeated exposure to a virus, amoebas carrying a virus, drugs, Haiti, voodoo, Flagyl, constant bouts of amebiasis, hepatitis A and B, syphilis, gonorrhea.

I have talked with the leading doctors treating us. One said to me, "If I knew in 1981 what I know now, I would never have become involved with this disease." Another said, "The thing that upsets me the most in all of this is that at any given moment one of my patients is in the hospital and something is going on with him that I don't understand. And it's destroying me because there's some craziness going on in him that's destroying him." A third said to me, "I'm very depressed. A doctor's job is to make patients well. And I can't. Too many of my patients die."

After almost two years of an epidemic, there still are no answers. After almost two years of an epidemic, the cause of AIDS remains unknown. After almost two years of an epidemic, there is no cure.

Hospitals are now so filled with AIDS patients that there is often a waiting period of up to a month before admission, no matter how sick you are. And, once in, patients are now more and more being treated like lepers as hospital staffs become increasingly worried that AIDS is infectious.

Suicides are now being reported of men who would rather die than face such medical uncertainty, such uncertain therapies, such hospital treatment, and the appalling statistic that 86 percent of all serious AIDS cases die after three years' time.

If all of this had been happening to any other community for two long years, there would have been, long ago, such an outcry from that community and all its members that the government of this city and this country would not know what had hit them.

Why isn't every gay man in this city so scared shitless that he is screaming for action? Does every gay man in New York *want* to die?

Let's talk about a few things specifically.

■ Let's talk about which gay men get AIDS.

No matter what you've heard, there is no single profile for all AIDS victims. There are drug users and non-drug users. There are the truly promiscuous and the almost monogamous. There are reported cases of single-contact infection.

All it seems to take is the one wrong fuck. That's not promiscuity—that's bad luck.

■ Let's talk about AIDS happening in straight people.

We have been hearing from the beginning of this epidemic that it was only a question of time before the straight community came down with AIDS, and that when that happened AIDS would suddenly be high on all agendas for funding and research and then we would finally be looked after and all would then be well.

I myself thought, when AIDS occurred in the first baby, that would be the breakthrough point. It was. For one day the media paid an enormous amount of attention. And that was it, kids.

There have been no confirmed cases of AIDS in straight, white, non-intravenous-drug-using, middle-class Americans.

The only confirmed straights struck down by AIDS are members of groups just as disenfranchised as gay men: intravenous drug users, Haitians, eleven hemophiliacs (up from eight), black and Hispanic babies, and wives or partners of IV drug users and bisexual men.

If there have been—and there may have been—any cases in straight, white, non-intravenous-drug-using, middle-class Americans, the Centers for Disease Control isn't telling anyone about them. When pressed, the CDC says there are "a number of cases that don't fall into any of the other categories." The CDC says it's impossible to fully investigate most of these "other category" cases; most of them are dead. The CDC also tends not to believe living, white, middle-class male victims when they say they're straight, or female victims when they say their husbands are straight and don't take drugs.

Why isn't AIDS happening to more straights? Maybe it's because gay men don't have sex with them.

Of all serious AIDS cases, 72.4 percent are in gay and bisexual men.

■ Let's talk about "surveillance."

The Centers for Disease Control is charged by our government to fully monitor all epidemics and unusual diseases.

To learn something from an epidemic, you have to keep records and statistics. Statistics come from interviewing victims and getting as much information from them as you can. Before they die. To get the best information, you have to ask the right questions.

There have been so many AIDS victims that the CDC is no longer able to get to them fast enough. It has given up. (The CDC also had been using a questionnaire that was fairly insensitive to the lives of gay men, and thus the data collected from its early study of us have been disputed by gay epidemiologists. The National Institutes of Health is also fielding a very naïve questionnaire.)

Important, vital case histories are now being lost because of this cessation of CDC interviewing. This is a woeful waste with as terrifying implications for us as the alarming rise in case numbers and doctors finally admitting they don't know what's going on. As each man dies, as one or both sets of men who had interacted with each other come down with AIDS, yet more information that might reveal patterns of transmissibility is not being monitored and collected and studied. We are being denied perhaps the easiest and fastest research tool available at this moment.

It will require at least $200,000 to prepare a new questionnaire to study the next important question that must be answered: *How* is AIDS being transmitted? (In which bodily fluids, by which sexual behaviors, in what social environments?)

For months the CDC has been asked to begin such preparations for continued surveillance. The CDC is stretched to its limits and is dreadfully underfunded for what it's being asked, in all areas, to do.

■ Let's talk about various forms of treatment.

It is very difficult for a patient to find out which hospital to go to or which doctor to go to or which mode of treatment to attempt.

Hospitals and doctors are reluctant to reveal how well they're doing with each type of treatment. They may, if you press them, give you a general idea. Most will not show you their precise numbers of how many patients are doing well on what and how many failed to respond adequately.

Because of the ludicrous requirements of the medical journals, doctors are prohibited from revealing publicly the specific data they are gathering from their treatments of our bodies. Doctors and hospitals need money for research, and this money (from the National Institutes of Health, from cancer research funding organizations, from rich patrons) comes based on the performance of their work (i.e., their tabulations of their results of their treatment of our bodies); this performance is written up as "papers" that must be submitted to and accepted by such "distinguished" medical publications as the *New England Journal of Medicine*. Most of these "distinguished" publications, however, will not publish anything that has been spoken of, leaked, announced, or intimated publicly in advance. Even after acceptance, the doctors must hold their tongues until the article is actually published. Dr. Bijan Safai of Sloan-Kettering has been waiting over six months for the *New England Journal*, which has accepted his interferon study, to publish it. Until that happens, he is only permitted to speak in the most general terms of how interferon is or is not working.

Priorities in this area appear to be peculiarly out of kilter at this moment of life or death.

■   Let's talk about hospitals.
Everybody's full up, fellows. No room in the inn.
Part of this is simply overcrowding. Part of this is cruel.
Sloan-Kettering still enforces a regulation from pre-AIDS days that only one dermatology patient per week can be admitted to that hospital. (Kaposi's sarcoma falls under dermatology at Sloan-Kettering.) But Sloan-Kettering is also the second-largest treatment center for AIDS patients in New York. You can be near death and still not get into Sloan-Kettering.

Additionally, Sloan-Kettering (and the Food and Drug Administration) requires patients to receive their initial shots of interferon while they are hospitalized. A lot of men want to try interferon at Sloan-Kettering before they try chemotherapy elsewhere.

It's not hard to see why there's such a waiting list to get into Sloan-Kettering.

Most hospital staffs are still so badly educated about AIDS that they don't know much about it, except that they've heard it's infectious. (There still have been no cases in hospital staff or among the very doctors who have been treating AIDS victims for two years.) Hence, as I said earlier, AIDS patients are often treated like lepers.

For various reasons, I would not like to be a patient at the Veterans Administration Hospital on East 24th Street or at New York Hospital. (Incidents involving AIDS patients at these two hospitals have been reported in news stories in the *Native*.)

I believe it falls to this city's Department of Health, under Commissioner David Sencer, and the Health and Hospitals Corporation, under Commissioner Stanley Brezenoff, to educate this city, its citizens, and its hospital workers about all areas of a public health emergency. Well, they have done an appalling job of educating our citizens, our hospital workers, and even, in some instances, our doctors. Almost everything this city knows about AIDS has come to it, in one way or another, through Gay Men's Health Crisis. And that includes television programs, magazine articles, radio commercials, newsletters, health-recommendation brochures, open forums, and sending speakers everywhere, including—when asked—into hospitals. If three out of four AIDS cases were occurring in straights instead of in gay men, you can bet all hospitals and their staffs would know what was happening. And it would be this city's Health Department and Health and Hospitals Corporation that would be telling them.

■ Let's talk about what gay tax dollars are buying for gay men.

Now we're arriving at the truly scandalous.

For over a year and a half the National Institutes of Health has been "reviewing" which from among some $55 million worth of grant applications for AIDS research money it will eventually fund.

It's not even a question of NIH having to ask Congress for money. It's already there. Waiting. NIH has almost $8 million already appropriated that it has yet to release into usefulness.

There is no question that if this epidemic was happening to the straight, white, non-intravenous-drug-using middle class, that money would have been put into use almost two years ago, when the first alarming signs of this epidemic were noticed by Dr. Alvin Friedman-Kien and Dr. Linda Laubenstein at New York University Hospital.

During the first *two weeks* of the Tylenol scare, the United States Government spent $10 million to find out what was happening.

Every hospital in New York that's involved in AIDS research has used up every bit of the money it could find for researching AIDS while waiting for NIH grants to come through. These hospitals have been working on AIDS for up to two years and are now desperate for replenishing funds. Important studies that began last year, such as Dr. Michael Lange's at St. Luke's-Roosevelt, are now going under for lack of money. Important leads that were and are developing cannot be pursued. (For instance, few hospitals can afford plasmapheresis machines, and few patients can afford this experimental treatment either, since few insurance policies will cover the $16,600 bill.) New York University Hospital, the largest treatment

center for AIDS patients in the world, has had its grant application pending at NIH for a year and a half. Even if the application is successful, the earliest time that NYU could receive any
money would be late summer.

The NIH would probably reply that it's foolish just to throw
money away, that that hasn't worked before. And, NIH would
say, if nobody knows what's happening, what's to study?

Any good administrator with half a brain could survey the
entire AIDS mess and come up with twenty leads that merit
further investigation. I could do so myself. In any research, in
any investigation, you have to start somewhere. You can't just
not start anywhere at all.

But then, AIDS is happening mostly to gay men, isn't it?

All of this is indeed ironic. For within AIDS, as most researchers have been trying to convey to the NIH, perhaps may
reside the answer to the question of what it is that causes
cancer itself. If straights had more brains, or were less bigoted
against gays, they would see that, as with hepatitis B, gay men
are again doing their suffering for them, revealing this disease
to them. They can use us as guinea pigs to discover the cure for
AIDS before it hits them, which most medical authorities are
still convinced will be happening shortly in increasing numbers.

(As if it had not been malevolent enough, the NIH is now,
for unspecified reasons, also turning away AIDS patients from
its hospital in Bethesda, Maryland. The hospital, which had
been treating anyone and everyone with AIDS free of charge,
now will only take AIDS patients if they fit into their current
investigating protocol. Whatever that is. The NIH publishes
"papers," too.)

Gay men pay taxes just like everyone else. NIH money
should be paying for our research just like everyone else's. We
desperately need something from our government to save our
lives, and we're not getting it.

■   Let's talk about health insurance and welfare problems.

Many of the ways of treating AIDS are experimental, and
many health insurance policies do not cover most of them. Blue
Cross is particularly bad about accepting anything unusual.

Many serious victims of AIDS have been unable to qualify

for welfare or disability or social security benefits. There are increasing numbers of men unable to work and unable to claim welfare because AIDS is not on the list of qualifying disability illnesses. (Immune deficiency is an acceptable determining factor for welfare among children, but not adults. Figure that one out.) There are also increasing numbers of men unable to pay their rent, men thrown out on the street with nowhere to live and no money to live with, and men who have been asked by roommates to leave because of their illnesses. And men with serious AIDS are being fired from certain jobs.

The horror stories in this area, of those suddenly found destitute, of those facing this illness with insufficient insurance, continue to mount. (One man who'd had no success on other therapies was forced to beg from his friends the $16,600 he needed to try, as a last resort, plasmapheresis.)

■ Finally, let's talk about our mayor, Ed Koch.

Our mayor, Ed Koch, appears to have chosen, for whatever reason, not to allow himself to be perceived by the non-gay world as visibly helping us in this emergency.

Repeated requests to meet with him have been denied us. Repeated attempts to have him make a very necessary public announcement about this crisis and public health emergency have been refused by his staff.

I sometimes think he doesn't know what's going on. I sometimes think that, like some king who has been so long on his throne he's lost touch with his people, Koch is so protected and isolated by his staff that he is unaware of what fear and pain we're in. No *human* being could otherwise continue to be so useless to his suffering constituents. When I was allowed a few moments with him at a party for outgoing Cultural Affairs Commissioner (and Gay Men's Health Crisis Advisory Board Member) Henry Geldzahler, I could tell from his responses that Mayor Koch had not been well briefed on AIDS or what is happening in his city. When I started to fill him in, I was pulled away by an aide, who said, "Your time is up."

I could see our mayor relatively blameless in his shameful secreting of himself from our need of him in this time of epidemic—except for one fact. Our mayor thinks so little of us that

he has assigned as his "liaison" to the gay community a man
of such appalling insensitivity to our community and its needs
that I am ashamed to say he is a homosexual. His name is Herb
Rickman, and for a while our mayor saw fit to have Rickman
serve as liaison to the Hasidic Jewish community, too. Hasidic
Jews hate gays. Figure out a mayor who would do that to you.

To continue to allow Herb Rickman to represent us in City
Hall will, in my view, only bring us closer to death.

When I denounced Rickman at a recent gay Community
Council meeting, I received a resounding ovation. He is almost
universally hated by virtually every gay organization in New
York. Why, then, have we all allowed this man to shit on us so,
to refuse our phone calls, to scream at us hysterically, to slam
down telephones, to threaten us, to tease us with favors that
are not delivered, to keep us waiting hours for an audience, to
lie to us—in short, to humiliate us so? He would not do this to
black or Jewish leaders. And they would not take it from him
for one minute. Why, why, why do we allow him to do it to us?
And he, a homosexual!

One can only surmise that our mayor wants us treated this
way.

My last attempt at communication with Herb Rickman was
on January 23rd [1983], when, after several days of his not
returning my phone calls, I wrote to him that the mayor continued to ignore our crisis at his peril. And I state here and now
that if Mayor Ed Koch continues to remain invisible to us and
to ignore us in this era of mounting death, I swear I shall do
everything in my power to see that he never wins elective office
again.

Rickman would tell you that the mayor is concerned, that he
has established an "Inter-Departmental Task Force"—and, as
a member of it, I will tell you that this Task Force is just lip
service and a waste of everyone's time. It hasn't even met for
two months. (Health Commissioner David Sencer had his gall-
stones out.)

On October 28th, 1982, Mayor Koch was implored to make
a public announcement about our emergency. If he had done so
then, and if he was only to do so now, the following would be
put into action:

1. The community at large would be alerted (you would be amazed at how many people, including gay men, still don't know enough about the AIDS danger).

2. Hospital staffs and public assistance offices would also be alerted and their education commenced.

3. The country, President Reagan, and the National Institutes of Health, as well as Congress, would be alerted, and these constitute the most important ears of all.

If the mayor doesn't think it's important enough to talk up AIDS, none of these people is going to, either.

The Mayor of New York has an enormous amount of power—when he wants to use it. When he wants to help his people. With the failure yet again of our civil rights bill, I'd guess our mayor doesn't want to use his power to help us.

With his silence on AIDS, the Mayor of New York is helping to kill us.

■ ■ ■

I am sick of our electing officials who in no way represent us. I am sick of our stupidity in believing candidates who promise us everything for our support and promptly forget us and insult us after we have given them our votes. Koch is the prime example, but not the only one. Daniel Patrick Moynihan isn't looking very good at this moment, either. Moynihan was requested by gay leaders to publicly ask Margaret Heckler at her confirmation hearing for Secretary of Health and Human Services if she could be fair to gays in view of her voting record of definite anti-gay bias. (Among other horrors, she voted to retain the sodomy law in Washington, D.C., at Jerry Falwell's request.) Moynihan refused to ask this question, as he has refused to meet with us about AIDS, despite our repeated requests. Margaret Heckler will have important jurisdiction over the CDC, over the NIH, over the Public Health Service, over the Food and Drug Administration—indeed, over all areas of AIDS concerns. Thank you, Daniel Patrick Moynihan. I am sick of our not realizing we have enough votes to defeat these people, and I am sick of our not electing our own openly gay officials in the first place. Moynihan doesn't even have an openly gay person on his staff, and he represents the city with the largest gay population in America.

I am sick of closeted gay doctors who won't come out to help us fight to rectify any of what I'm writing about. Doctors—the very letters "M.D."—have enormous clout, particularly when they fight in groups. Can you imagine what gay doctors could accomplish, banded together in a network, petitioning local and federal governments, straight colleagues, and the American Medical Association? I am sick of the passivity or nonparticipation or halfhearted protestation of all the gay medical associations (American Physicians for Human Rights, Bay Area Physicians for Human Rights, Gay Psychiatrists of New York, etc., etc.), and particularly our own New York Physicians for Human Rights, a group of 175 of our gay doctors who have, as a group, done *nothing.* You can count on one hand the number of our doctors who have really worked for *us.*

I am sick of the *Advocate,* one of this country's largest gay publications, which has yet to quite acknowledge that there's anything going on. That newspaper's recent AIDS issue was so innocuous you'd have thought all we were going through was little worse than a rage of the latest designer flu. And their own associate editor, Brent Harris, died from AIDS. Figure that one out.

With the exception of the *New York Native* and a few, very few, other gay publications, the gay press has been useless. If we can't get our own papers and magazines to tell us what's really happening to us, and this negligence is added to the negligent non-interest of the straight press (*The New York Times* took a leisurely year and a half between its major pieces, and the *Village Voice* took a year and a half to write anything at all), how are we going to get the word around that we're dying? Gay men in smaller towns and cities everywhere must be educated, too. Has the *Times* or the *Advocate* told you that twenty-nine cases have been reported from Paris?

I am sick of gay men who won't support gay charities. Go give your bucks to straight charities, fellows, while we die. Gay Men's Health Crisis is going crazy trying to accomplish everything it does—printing and distributing hundreds of thousands of educational items, taking care of several hundred AIDS victims (some of them straight) in and out of hospitals, arranging community forums and speakers all over this country, getting media attention, fighting bad hospital care, on and on and on, fighting for you and us in two thousand ways, *and* trying to sell 17,600 Circus tickets, too. Is the Red Cross doing this for you? Is the American Cancer Society? Your college alumni fund? The United Jewish Appeal? Catholic Charities? The United Way? The Lenox Hill Neighborhood Association, or any of the other fancy straight charities for which faggots put on black ties and dance at the Plaza? The National Gay Task Force—our only hope for national leadership, with its new and splendid leader, Virginia Apuzzo—which is spending more and more time fighting for the AIDS issue, is broke. Senior Action in a Gay Environment and Gay Men's Health Crisis are, within a few months, going to be without office space they can afford, and thus will be out on the street. The St. Mark's Clinic, held together by some of the few devoted gay doctors in this city who aren't interested in becoming rich, lives in constant terror of even higher rent and eviction. This community is desperate for the services these organizations are providing for it. And these organizations are all desperate for money, which is certainly not coming from straight people or President Reagan or Mayor Koch. (If every gay man within a 250-mile radius of Manhattan isn't in Madison Square Garden on the night of April 30th to help Gay Men's Health Crisis make enough money to get through the next horrible year of fighting against AIDS, I shall lose all hope that we have any future whatsoever.)

I am sick of closeted gays. It's 1983 already, guys, when are you going to come out? By 1984 you could be dead. Every gay man who is unable to come forward now and fight to save his own life is truly helping to kill the rest of us. There is only one thing that's going to save some of us, and this is *numbers* and pressure and our being perceived as united and a threat. As more and more of my friends die, I have less and less sympathy for men who are afraid their mommies will find out or afraid their bosses will find out or afraid their fellow doctors or professional associates will find out. Unless we can generate, visibly, numbers, masses, we are going to die.

I am sick of everyone in this community who tells me to stop creating a panic. How many of us have to die before *you* get

scared off your ass and into action? Aren't 195 dead New Yorkers enough? Every straight person who is knowledgeable about
the AIDS epidemic can't understand why gay men aren't
marching on the White House. Over and over again I hear from
them, "Why aren't you guys doing anything?" Every politician
I have spoken to has said to me confidentially, "You guys aren't
making enough noise. Bureaucracy only responds to pressure."

I am sick of people who say "it's no worse than statistics for
smokers and lung cancer" or "considering how many homosexuals there are in the United States, AIDS is really statistically
affecting only a very few." That would wash if there weren't
164 cases in twenty-eight days. That would wash if case numbers hadn't jumped from 41 to 1,112 in eighteen months. That
would wash if cases in one city—New York—hadn't jumped to
cases in fifteen countries and thirty-five states (up from thirty-
four last week). That would wash if cases weren't coming in at
more than four a day nationally and over two a day locally. That
would wash if the mortality rate didn't start at 38 percent the
first year of diagnosis and climb to a grotesque 86 percent after
three years. Get your stupid heads out of the sand, you turkeys!

I am sick of guys who moan that giving up careless sex until
this blows over is worse than death. How can they value life so
little and cocks and asses so much? Come with me, guys, while
I visit a few of our friends in Intensive Care at NYU. Notice the
looks in their eyes, guys. They'd give up sex forever if you
could promise them life.

I am sick of guys who think that all being gay means is sex
in the first place. I am sick of guys who can only think with their
cocks.

I am sick of "men" who say, "We've got to keep quiet or
they will do such and such." *They* usually means the straight
majority, the "Moral" Majority, or similarly perceived representatives of *them*. Okay, you "men"—be my guests: You can
march off now to the gas chambers; just get right in line.

We shall always have enemies. Nothing we can ever do will
remove them. Southern newspapers and Jerry Falwell's publications are already printing editorials proclaiming AIDS as
God's deserved punishment on homosexuals. So what? Nasty
words make poor little sissy pansy wilt and die?

And I am very sick and saddened by every gay man who

does not get behind this issue totally and with commitment—to fight for his life.

■ ■ ■

I don't want to die. I can only assume you don't want to die. Can we fight together?

For the past few weeks, about fifty community leaders and organization representatives have been meeting at Beth Simchat Torah, the gay synagogue, to prepare action. We call ourselves the AIDS Network. We come from all areas of health concern: doctors, social workers, psychologists, psychiatrists, nurses; we come from Gay Men's Health Crisis, from the National Gay Health Education Foundation, from New York Physicians for Human Rights, the St. Mark's Clinic, the Gay Men's Health Project; we come from the gay synagogue, the Gay Men's Chorus, from the Greater Gotham Business Council, SAGE, Lambda Legal Defense, Gay Fathers, the Christopher Street Festival Committee, Dignity, Integrity; we are lawyers, actors, dancers, architects, writers, citizens; we come from many component organizations of the Gay and Lesbian Community Council.

We have a leader. Indeed, for the first time our community appears to have a true leader. Her name is Virginia Apuzzo, she is head of the National Gay Task Force, and, as I have said, so far she has proved to be magnificent.

The AIDS Network has sent a letter to Mayor Koch. It contains twelve points that are urged for his consideration and action.

This letter to Mayor Koch also contains the following paragraph:

> It must be stated at the outset that the gay community is growing increasingly aroused and concerned and angry. Should our avenues to the mayor of our city and the members of the Board of Estimate not be available, it is our feeling that the level of frustration is such that it will manifest itself in a manner heretofore not associated with this community and the gay population at large. It should be stated, too, at the outset, that as of February 25th, there were 526 cases of serious AIDS in New York's

metropolitan area and 195 deaths (and 1,112 cases nationally and 418 deaths) and it is the sad and sorry fact that
most gay men in our city now have close friends and lovers
who have either been stricken with or died from this disease. It is against this background that this letter is addressed. It is this issue that has, ironically, united our
community in a way not heretofore thought possible.

Further, a number of AIDS Network members have been
studying civil disobedience with one of the experts from Dr.
Martin Luther King's old team. We are learning how. Gay men
are the strongest, toughest people I know. We are perhaps
shortly to get an opportunity to show it.

I'm sick of hearing that Mayor Koch doesn't respond to
pressures and threats from the disenfranchised, that he walks
away from confrontations. Maybe he does. But we have *tried*
to make contact with him, we are *dying*, so what other choice
but confrontation has he left us?

I hope we don't have to conduct sit-ins or tie up traffic or get
arrested. I hope our city and our country will start to do something to help start saving us. But it is time for us to be perceived
for what we truly are: an angry community and a strong community, and therefore *a threat*. Such are the realities of politics. Nationally we are 24 million strong, which is more than
there are Jews or blacks or Hispanics in this country.

I want to make a point about what happens if we *don't* get
angry about AIDS. There are the obvious losses, of course:
Little of what I've written about here is likely to be rectified
with the speed necessary to help the growing number of victims. But something worse will happen, and is already happening. Increasingly, we are being *blamed* for AIDS, for this
epidemic; we are being called its perpetrators, through our
blood, through our "promiscuity," through just being the gay
men so much of the rest of the world has learned to hate. We
can point out until we are blue in the face that we are not the
cause of AIDS but its victims, that AIDS has landed among us
first, as it could have landed among them first. But other frightened populations are going to drown out these truths by playing on the worst bigoted fears of the straight world, and send
the status of gays right back to the Dark Ages. Not all Jews

are blamed for Meyer Lansky, Rabbis Bergman and Kahane, or for money-lending. All Chinese aren't blamed for the recent Seattle slaughters. But all gays are blamed for John Gacy, the North American Man/Boy Love Association, and AIDS.

Enough. I am told this is one of the longest articles the *Native* has ever run. I hope I have not been guilty of saying ineffectively in five thousand words what I could have said in five: we must fight to live.

I am angry and frustrated almost beyond the bound my skin and bones and body and brain can encompass. My sleep is tormented by nightmares and visions of lost friends, and my days are flooded by the tears of funerals and memorial services and seeing my sick friends. How many of us must die before *all* of us living fight back?

I know that unless I fight with every ounce of my energy I will hate myself. I hope, I pray, I implore you to feel the same.

I am going to close by doing what Dr. Ron Grossman did at GMHC's second Open Forum last November at Julia Richman High School. He listed the names of the patients he had lost to AIDS. Here is a list of twenty dead men I knew:

Nick Rock

Rick Wellikoff

Jack Nau

Shelly

Donald Krintzman

Jerry Green

Michael Maletta

Paul Graham

Toby

Harry Blumenthal

Stephen Sperry

Brian O'Hara

Barry

David

Jeffrey Croland

Z.

David Jackson

Tony Rappa

Robert Christian

Ron Doud

And one more, who will be dead by the time these words appear in print.

If we don't act immediately, then we face our approaching doom.

■ ■ ■

Volunteers Needed for Civil Disobedience

It is necessary that we have a pool of at least three thousand people who are prepared to participate in demonstrations of civil disobedience. Such demonstrations might include sit-ins or traffic tie-ups. All participants must be prepared to be arrested. I am asking every gay person and every gay organization to canvass all friends and members and make a count of the total number of people you can provide toward this pool of three thousand.

Let me know how many people you can be counted on providing. Just include the number of people; you don't have to send actual names—you keep that list yourself. And include your own phone numbers. *Start these lists now.*

L.K.

This essay managed to create quite a stir, but more so in cities other than New York. It was reprinted in almost every major gay newspaper across the country. I told the Board of GMHC that I was writing it, and they told me to put in the disclaimer that I was speaking for myself and not our organization. When it appeared, they hated it.

The appeal for volunteers for civil disobedience was not successful. A group of about fifty managed to coalesce and meet for instruction with a straight black man who had worked with Martin Luther King, Jr. We called ourselves the AIDS Network Public Events Committee. Such a small number didn't augur well. But, as will be seen, it proved to be sufficient.

Although this article is dated after the letter to the mayor that follows, it's placed first for background. The repercussions from the letter to the mayor were to lead to the final break in my affiliation with Gay Men's Health Crisis, which this present article, along with all my media appearances, greatly exacerbated.

The AIDS Network Letter to Mayor Koch

3 March 83

Hon. Edward I. Koch
Mayor, City of New York
City Hall
New York, New York 10007

Dear Mayor Koch,

The AIDS Network, a gay community group of concerned health-care professionals, doctors, psychiatrists, psychologists, social workers, representatives of (including but not limited to) Gay Men's Health Crisis, National Gay Health Education Foundation, the Gay Synagogue, National Gay Task Force, Greater Gotham Business Council, New York Physicians for Human Rights, St. Mark's Clinic, and the Gay and Lesbian Community Council and all of its component organizations—having met together because of their growing concern over the alarming rise of serious cases of AIDS and the high mortality rate therefrom, and the general feeling that the City of New York, where 56.5 percent of all serious cases of AIDS cases are occurring, is not perceived as working swiftly enough to fight this fast-growing epidemic on all fronts—addresses the following requests to the Mayor of our City and to the Board of Estimate, along with the fervent plea that an immediate meeting be scheduled for a personal presentation.

It must be stated at the outset that the gay community is growing increasingly aroused and concerned and angry. Should our avenues to the Mayor of our City and the members of the Board of Estimate not be available, it is our feeling that the level of frustration is such that it will manifest itself in a manner heretofore not associated with this community and the gay population at large. It should be stated, too, at the outset, that as of February 25th, there were 526 cases of serious AIDS in New York's metropolitan area and 195 deaths, and it is the sad and sorry fact that most gay men in our city now have close friends and lovers who have either been stricken with or died from this disease. It is against this background that this letter is addressed. It is this issue that has, ironically, united our community in a way not heretofore thought possible.

The following points are urged upon the Mayor for his consideration and action:

1. PUBLIC ANNOUNCEMENT: The first and primary point is that the Mayor *publicly* pronounce to this City that it is in a state of extreme public health emergency. This announcement should be made to the press and all media so that its import can be immediately responded to. It is imperative that such an announcement be made and is indeed placed first among our demands since, in making this announcement, the Mayor is in fact placing into motion action on all the following points requiring immediate action.

2. EDUCATION: It is imperative that all sectors of the community be educated about the present emergency, including the populations at risk, which, at present, include gay men, Haitians, those populations liable to intravenous drug use, and hemophiliacs. It is imperative that such education inform people that the stricken communities not be stigmatized as the cause of AIDS, for they truly are the victims of this epidemic.

Health-care and hospital workers and mental-health providers of social and all public assistance services must also be educated immediately. It must be borne in mind that at present many hospital workers are simply not familiar with the problems of AIDS, how to care for AIDS patients, and the question of contagion. This applies to both city and voluntary hospitals. The number of complaints arising from all hospitals of improper patient care is rising.

3. CITY AIDS COORDINATOR AND OFFICE: That the Mayor establish the paid position of City AIDS Coordinator, together with a City AIDS Coordination Office. The appointment of this Coordinator is to be made in consultation with the stricken communities. The job of this Coordinator and this Office would be to oversee all AIDS activities and to be knowledgeable of everything that is transpiring in each department and organization in the AIDS Network.

4. INTER-DEPARTMENTAL TASK FORCE: MAYOR'S OFFICE REPRESENTATIVE: That there be a member of the Mayor's immediate staff appointed to join the monthly Inter-Departmental Task Force that the Mayor has already established and presently under the Chairmanship of Health Commissioner David Sencer.

5. INTER-DEPARTMENTAL TASK FORCE: BOARD OF ESTIMATE REPRESENTATIVES: That each member of the Board of Estimate have a representative on this Inter-Departmental Task Force.

6. INTER-DEPARTMENTAL TASK FORCE: MEETINGS: That this Inter-Departmental Task Force meet on a more regular basis and be empowered to achieve results.

7. ACCELERATION OF RESEARCH MONIES: That the Mayor contact the President of the United States personally, as well as the Governor of this State, and Congress, and urge that all use every power to accelerate the release of research monies already appropriated by the National Institutes of Health but still not granted to the many local and national doctors, hospitals, and laboratories clamoring to study AIDS. It is imperative that each of these parties be asked to locate and identify all discretion-

ary funds that might be immediately put to use to fight AIDS. All major New York hospitals and research facilities have been waiting in excess of one year for much needed monies to replenish their long-ago-depleted research funds.

8. RESEARCH: That the Mayor see to it that AIDS be represented in the new supplemental budget that the President will submit to Congress, and that the Mayor see to it that, in view of all new recent developments, the National Institutes of Health be funded to immediately process a second call of grant requests.

And that these funds be adequate to provide and support scientific investigation for: epidemiological research to determine risk factors and transmissibility, and to establish comprehensive national disease surveillance programs; socio-medical research to develop measures to assess social behavior, patterns of intimate contact, and characteristics of social support; immunological research to improve the medical and psycho-social treatment of patients. The combined goals of this research are to define and control this disorder. All of this is to be done in consultation and contact with the AIDS Scientific Review Board already established in this City.

9. IMMEDIATE REESTABLISHMENT OF SURVEILLANCE OF THE STRICKEN COMMUNITIES: That efforts be made to urge the Centers for Disease Control to join with Gay Men's Health Crisis and the AIDS Scientific Advisory Board in reestablishing epidemiological surveillance of, particularly, the gay community AIDS victims, which has presently been discontinued. This is imperative work that is not being done. An invaluable research tool is not being utilized.

10. PUBLIC ASSISTANCE AND PRIVATE INSURANCE CLAIMS: That the immense problems being encountered by patients and victims of AIDS in the areas of public assistance and social security and disability and Medicaid be addressed. There are increasing numbers of people unable to work and unable to claim various forms of welfare because AIDS is not on the list of qualifying disability illnesses. That the State Insurance Commission

also investigate private insurance companies' practices in rejecting claims for AIDS patients and victims.

11. SIGNIFICANT OTHERS: That a policy be adopted wherein and whereby patients are allowed to identify who their significant others are. Hospitals and health-care facilities should be advised that gay people consider lovers, partners, and friends as members of their primary family, and these should be judged as such and not refused admission to patients as not being family members, spouses, or blood relatives.

12. HEALTH-CARE EMERGENCY SPACE: A public health emergency requires space to administer to its problems, and Gay Men's Health Crisis, Inc., at present the organization most actively involved in tending to the many problems in the communities at highest risks, is without adequate space for its office and for the many patient services programs it performs, including Crisis Intervention Counseling, Individual Therapy and Group Support Therapy for victims of AIDS, Kaposi's sarcoma cancer, and *Pneumocystis carinii* pneumonia, and maintenance of its extensive community education programs that have resulted in hundreds of thousands of items of instruction and recommendation.

While it is the space problem of Gay Men's Health Crisis that is of most pressing immediate concern, it is the hope of the gay and lesbian community that all of its vital social services, both pertaining to AIDS, in organizations such as GMHC and St. Mark's Clinic, and in other areas, such as, but not limited to, SAGE (Senior Action in a Gay Environment), the Fund for Human Dignity, Lambda Legal Defense, and gay religious organizations, for the first time find a home under one roof to form a Gay Community Center, such as exists in the cities of Los Angeles, Philadelphia, and Houston. The old high school on West 13th Street would be ideal for this purpose.

Finally and in summation, while we are eager to speak for all at-risk communities, these points represent the concerns of the gay community mainly, though an effort to form a coalition of all at-risk groups has been made. A face-to-face meeting with the Mayor is requested with all dispatch so that the above can be attended to in as swift a fashion as possible, and so that the period of suffering for those stricken can be alleviated with all similar speed.

The favor of an acknowledgment is requested within thirty days from this date.

T he AIDS Network was an ad hoc group that met, for several years, once a week at 8:00 A.M. It was formed by many who felt left out of GMHC, which unfortunately was gaining an "elitist" reputation. The remarkable fact about GMHC, that it was attracting many who had never participated in gay organizations or in anything having remotely to do with gay politics, worked against it in that many who had participated in the gay movement for years now felt disenfranchised and unwelcome at the most vital new center of gay activity. And these newcomers to "activism"—as it was becoming increasingly and tragically clear—were not "activists" at all; they were concerned citizens who wished to help quietly, in the pastoral sense. And so continued the concretizing of GMHC into its present state: that of a social service organization, rather than an advocacy one. While I supported the necessity for the former, I was passionately committed to the latter as well. GMHC, as far as I was concerned, was formed primarily to spread information and fight in every way to help the living keep living. And it was this fight to include my priorities in GMHC's agenda that I was losing, and was about to lose completely.

It was to the AIDS Network that these veterans of years of involvement in the gay movement came, as well as newcomers who shared their desires for more aggressive tactics of confrontation. I wrote the above letter with much input from those who attended an

emergency meeting I called. The letter was then signed
by representatives of some sixty gay organizations and
hand-delivered to the offices of the mayor and each member of the Board of Estimate. The mayor did not respond. On Sunday, April 10th, a very small group of
us—no more than twenty—picketed in torrential rain,
outside Lenox Hill Hospital, where the mayor was making an appearance at the historic AIDS Conference organized by Dr. Kevin Cahill (where he somehow
managed to induce appearances not only by the mayor
but by Cardinal Cooke as well, in addition to having a
statement from Senator Edward Kennedy read at the
opening).

This picketing was extensively televised locally, as
were the placards themselves, which included ones calling the mayor "blind" and "a coward" and one that said,
HEY, ED, COME OUT OF THE CLOSET AND HELP YOUR GAY
BROTHERS.

The very next morning, word was sent out from City
Hall that the mayor would finally meet with ten people
from the gay community.

When I arrived at the next meeting of the AIDS
Network, the ten people had already been chosen. Paul
Popham had, with the approval of GMHC's Board,
elected to take with him Mel Rosen, a graduate student
who was GMHC's part-time, volunteer, executive director.

I am not particularly proud of my subsequent behav-
ior, though I have come to understand it. I felt betrayed.
I had spent two years working full time to build GMHC.
I had called for the mayor's meeting and had arranged
the above petition. I told Paul that if I was not allowed
to attend, I would resign. He told me he had polled the
Board and they wished Mel to go. He said they were all
afraid I'd yell at the mayor and be an embarrassment.
I realized they wanted me to resign. That really hurt.
Petulantly, defensively, I resigned. Though I was implored by such gay leaders as Judge Richard Failla,
Virginia Apuzzo, and the late Peter Vogel, I stubbornly
refused to reconsider. Even when the AIDS Network

agreed to let me go as one of their representatives, I declined. I was furious and hurt and probably burned out. My friend Rodger McFarlane maintains that I was subconsciously preparing this break—that I wanted to write what was eventually to become my play *The Normal Heart*, and this was the only way I could allow myself to do so without feeling guilty.

Nevertheless, I did feel guilty, for quite some time, that I had so behaved. For many years I berated myself that, had I only stayed with GMHC, it would have included among its many activities the political-advocacy tasks that no one else was performing.

I was also to learn yet another lesson: When you are affiliated with an established organization, it's much easier to be taken seriously when talking to the media. Now I was disenfranchised, and I had lost my official soapbox.

Not one item of any substance was achieved at the mayor's meeting on April 20th. He listened, and did nothing. Matters remained as they were before. And as many of them still are now.

The Mark of Courage

It is now more than two years since AIDS entered our lives. Every one of us has learned more in these two years than ever before about what it means to be gay—in all ways, good and bad.

I am prouder now of gay people than ever. We have never been closer together as a community than we are now. We are learning how courageous we are. To oppression, homophobia, discrimination, self-hate, religions that don't want us, and families that think we're freaks, has now been added an epidemic that kills. We have to be courageous to live through all of this. Gay men and lesbians are the most courageous people I know.

Courage is a wonderful quality, one of the best. But how do we take it and make it work for us?

We've all learned a few hard lessons during these past two long years. One is that AIDS represents how badly we're served by our medical system.

* Gay Pride Day speech, June 26, 1983, delivered at parade rally. Published in the *New York Native,* Issue 67, July 4–17, 1983.

Another is that, as a community, so far we still have very little political power.

It has taken two long years to get Congress to consider AIDS funding. It has taken two long years for the National Institutes of Health to consider to whom to give funding. It has taken two long years to get the media to pay attention to AIDS. It has taken two long years to get *The New York Times* to write with any regularity about an epidemic that's occuring in its very own city. And it has taken two long years to get our very own mayor to timidly acknowledge that we have an emergency here.

Who knows how many more people will die needlessly because of this unconscionable tardiness?

The official rate of AIDS cases is now up to seven a day. This is the *official* figure; it is low. Because names of patients go onto lists that enter government computers, many patients and their doctors are now refusing to report their cases to the Centers for Disease Control, which is unable to guarantee confidentiality.

We must find ways of making sure these atrocities never, never happen again.

The White House is threatening to veto the supplemental budget that contains $12 million for AIDS. Reagan's men have specifically identified the AIDS funding allotment as being unnecessary. While I've been told this money will probably be found somewhere, the threatened veto only serves as another delay: Now the NIH will not release any more money for research until next October or November. These research grants are for three-year periods, so we're now looking at 1987 before these research reports on AIDS will be due.

Yes, we have to be courageous to live through all of this.

We have to be courageous as we wake up each day, as we wait for whatever we pray will be discovered to be discovered, and we continue to face the fact that *time is not on our side.*

I'd like to ask some questions.

Can we afford to have a New York gay community that is disorganized, lacking recognized and designated leaders who can speak for all of us? We must be able to send our best, brightest, smartest, cagiest, wisest to represent our side at various bargaining tables. We must not get bogged down with petty internal squabbles.

Can we afford to be disorganized nationally, with little political networking from city to city, from state to state?

Can we afford to be represented in Washington by only one lobbyist? Today, special-interest groups of every size and description support large staffs in Washington. We 24 million gay men and lesbians are going to have to dig into our pockets and pay for better and more extensive representation in our nation's capital, where so much of what affects us is decided. I am proud to cite the recent decision by the Board of Directors of Gay Men's Health Crisis to help establish a Washington lobby for AIDS with $40,000 of the dollars you have already contributed.

Can we afford to support just one gay charity or one gay issue? I call upon all gay organizations that seek money from the community to distribute their complete financial statements and a tally of their total paid-up membership—in other words, to be fiscally responsible. I call upon all members of the boards of directors of these organizations to retain their positions because of their skills and abilities, not for reasons of tokenism or friendship. It is essential that each organization be run by people who are the best that we can find, without regard to superfluous distinctions.

Can we afford to have such a bad relationship with the mayor of our very own city, whom we helped install in that very office? It took us nineteen months even to be heard. His office promised us space for AIDS patients and activities nine long months ago. We still have nothing. San Francisco's gay community has received $4 million from its mayor, and Houston has a gay vice-mayor. We don't even have a liaison from the mayor to the gay community on non-health issues who is available to us on any regular basis—much less one who does an acceptable job of representing our community.

Can we afford to be ignored by *The New York Times?* Yes, that paper is finally reporting about AIDS, but that's all that's being written about us. Any newspaper that refuses to report on the activities of one million of its constituent population is irresponsible. I'd like to suggest a twenty-four-hour-a-day, seven-days-a-week picket line outside the *New York Times* of-fices. We should carry neat placards: ONE MILLION GAY MEN AND LESBIANS WANT EQUAL TIME; ONE MILLION GAY MEN AND LESBIANS WANT TO BE CALLED GAY.

Can we afford any longer not to start our own Anti-Defama-tion League? This is an organization that the Jewish people started with only a handful of volunteers in 1913, "to stop the defamation of the Jewish people." In those days you could still see ads that demanded: "No dogs! No Jews!" You don't see that anymore because the Jews started an organization that pro-tests officially every single time anything anti-Semitic appears in public. It's time we started our own.

Can we afford duplication of energies and services? Do we need a Gay Men's Health Crisis and an AIDS Network and an ARC and a Gay Men With AIDS? Isn't there more strength in unity? Do we need both a National Gay Task Force and a Gay Rights National Lobby? If we do, could they not work together more effectively? And if we don't, could the boards of directors of these two organizations please join the rest of us in helping Virginia Apuzzo become the one truly national leader we so desperately need at this moment in history?

Can we afford not to have more support from our lesbian sisters at this time of crisis and as this crisis unites the gay male community?

Can we afford not to heal wounds and unite?

Can we afford not to have an openly gay member of the City Council? I support Bill Hirsch's excellent idea that all the money we collect at our local Human Rights Campaign Fund Dinner at the Waldorf stay right here in New York to find, nominate, campaign with, and elect our own openly gay candi-date.

Can we afford to continue living under the tyranny of beauty and muscles and big tits and big dicks and clonedom and youth? Can we afford not to begin working hard toward eroticizing intelligence, kindness, responsibility, devotion, achievement, respect—skills and qualities that are far more sexy, far more lasting, and far more important for our survival than big pecs and biceps and a washboard stomach?

Compared to what we have lived through these past two

years, to work on any or all of the above should not be as frightening.

I know that each and every one of us is scared and frightened in ways we've never been before. But let our fear not lead to denial, to going back into closets, to pretending. Let our fear give us extra courage. We are each our own masters.

To see the miraculous growth and ascending maturity of Gay Men's Health Crisis is to know what we are capable of doing when we put our minds and hearts into it. I would like to pay tribute here to the man who is president of that organization, Paul Popham. This community will never know the incredible extent of this man's devotion or how much it will be forever in his debt. He has learned, as we all are learning, as we all must learn, how to grow from day to day, each day at a time, each moment and bit by bit, so that we soon find ourselves able to perform feats we never imagined or dreamed we were capable of the day before.

On a personal note, I would like to apologize to any of the people dear to me whose feelings I may have bruised these past two years. I have been very much the angry man. It seems that in my frustration at seeing AIDS ignored for so long I just couldn't shut up. I have perhaps tried in too clumsy a fashion to hurry things along. I am by nature an impatient man.

But I am also a hopeful man. We have never felt the love of our fellow gay men and lesbians so much as in these past two years. This most dire emergency in our history is giving us the chance to fashion a new community.

With and from such love we can perform miracles. With and from such love our courage can take us to our future. With and from such love visions are formed and made reality. Each of us must put aside our fear and recognize the great courage within us, and take this courage and turn it into action. We must do nothing less now than remake the soul of our time. It is incumbent on us, the living, to do so, to ensure the future for our gay children, the millions and millions of proud gay men and lesbians who will follow us.

Solzhenitsyn warns us: "If we perish and lose this world, the fault will be ours alone." But we shall not lose it. We shall not perish. Our people are marching. Our people are courageous. Our people will survive.

I missed GMHC terribly. After such a long period of furious activity, constantly ringing phones, a mountain of problems waiting for solutions, and the sustaining comradeship of so many devoted fellow workers as we all aspired to make something happen, I now found myself alone at home, and feeling very much a pariah. One day there weren't enough hours in the day and the next day I had nothing to do. My phone hardly rang at all. I attended a few GMHC social functions, where I stood on one side of the room and the Board, only weeks before my closest friends, stood on the other. On one occasion, I commandeered the microphone in the DJ's booth of a bar where volunteers were being thanked with a party, and attempted to rouse them into action against the Board. "Tell them they made a mistake in letting me go. . . . Tell them they must fight harder and not be so timid and afraid. . . ." That sort of thing. When I emerged from the booth (I've been told that the whole episode was like something out of *Dr. Strangelove*), I was accosted by one of the volunteers, who started screaming at the top of his lungs that I was out to destroy GMHC. It dawned on me that now I couldn't even criticize this organization—which I had come to look upon as my child—and certainly not publicly, without inadvertently hurting it, perhaps stunting its growth in these early years of its development.

I wanted very much to come back to it (and I would later expend a great deal of useless energy in three separate attempts to get myself back on the Board), but I had made the decision that it was time to attempt to write something about my experiences since the epidemic began. It's not often that writers are so placed on the front line of history in the making, and I felt an obligation as well as the desire. I had earlier attempted to do so in a novel, but I'd found this form not immediate enough to convey the urgency of my feelings. Also, it had taken me three years to write *Faggots*, and I

wanted whatever I wrote to be out in the world as
quickly as possible. I also knew that no film company
would ever finance a movie about either AIDS or any
other subject remotely dealing with homosexuality.
That left only a play, and the only time I'd tried a play
before, I'd failed.

Well, I'd decided to go to Europe for the summer.
Perhaps in wandering about, the matter would sort itself out. And indeed it did. It was while I was in Germany, while visiting Dachau, that the thoughts began to
coalesce into what would shortly become my play *The
Normal Heart.*

Paul Popham and I had made peace with each other
shortly after the *Dr. Strangelove* episode. Somehow we
were still able to do that then. Our friendship and respect for each other was still able to survive our huge
differences in personality and style. He was a gentle,
quiet man, accustomed to the rigors and structures of
the corporate world and of the army, where he'd been
a Green Beret. He'd never had to work with a loose
cannon like me before, and I think most of the time I
was, for him, an exotic creature from another planet.
(He once told me he'd never met a Jew till college.) My
problem with him was of a different nature: I was half
in love with him, which he sensed and which made him
uncomfortable. (Straight men, I believe, don't usually
have these added problems in running their organizations.) This made it even more difficult for us to handle
our philosophical disagreements equably.

The performance of the Ringling Brothers Circus
that GMHC had bought out on April 30th was a huge
success. It was, up to that time, the biggest, most successful gay fund-raising event ever held, clearing over
a quarter of a million dollars. Leonard Bernstein walking across the length of Madison Square Garden in his
white dinner jacket to conduct the circus orchestra in
the national anthem, while eighteen thousand gay men
and their friends and families cheered, was one of the
most moving moments I have ever experienced. (*The
New York Times* did not report the occasion, a cruel

oversight that Abe Rosenthal was later shamed into apologizing for.) Paul generously announced to this crowd that I was leaving to take a rest, and that the Board wished to thank me for all my efforts. And the crowd cheered again, which I also will long remember.

I stayed on until June 26th, because I'd agreed to speak on Gay Pride Day. The version of my speech printed here is a bit more polite than some of my additions on the spot; I was gratified, when I called Mayor Koch "a heartless, selfish son of a bitch," that resounding cheers were heard again. I rushed to the airport and took a plane to Europe. I thought the bastard might be sending someone after me.

2,339 and Counting

I've been away from New York City for three months. I left after two miracles: the sold-out Circus benefit that Gay Men's Health Crisis sponsored in Madison Square Garden and the biggest Gay Pride Day parade New York gay people and their friends ever marched in together. Eighteen thousand at the first and many hundreds of thousands at the second. I was proud to be gay when I left New York. I had never seen the New York gay community so visibly together. The epidemic of AIDS had, miraculously and ironically, brought us together like the English at Dunkirk.

How could so much progress have evaporated so quickly?

I return to New York to find much of the New York gay community back at its petty bickerings, at the mercy of loud-mouth do-nothings murderously tying up what passes for political process among our disparate groups. I return to find Gay Men's Health Crisis—for two long and woeful years the only AIDS game in town for accurate information, for a list of social services that matches the Red Cross, for providing loving and supportive care to over four hundred patients—suddenly the

* *Village Voice*, October 4, 1983.

butt of outrageous and bitchy criticism. What should be cherished and supported by this community as a prideful treasure—and believe me, all of you gay men who are open to the possibility of contracting AIDS, there is no one else in this city who gives or cares much for us—has suddenly become the community's newest, most fashionable victim of badmouth. I returned to find GMHC's next vital fund-raiser, the October 1st Rodeo at Madison Square Garden, less than one-third sold out.

I return to find something else going on, just as bad and just as dangerous. Somehow there are waves of rumor that the epidemic is waning, that figures have slowed down, that, as in some fairy tale, we're all on our way to a happy ending and we can now return to apathy and closetry.

How can we be so dumb and blind and ignorant? In March, I wrote an article for the *New York Native* called "1,112 and Counting." Six months later there are more than twice as many cases in our country—2,339. Of these, 945 are dead. New York City is the home of over 40 percent of all victims—975, with 392 dead. (In March, New York figures were 526 cases and 195 dead.)

In June, 67 new cases were reported in this city; in July, 88 new cases were reported in this city; in August, 102 new cases were reported in this city. (Back in March, there were 56.) How can anyone believe things are getting better?

Almost three out of four cases still occur in sexually active gay men. "Sexually active" is defined as having sex once (i.e., the opposite of sexually inactive). The early profile of extreme promiscuity among victims is no longer accurate. A nun in Haiti has died from AIDS after having had sex only once in her life.

(Women now account for 151 cases, 59 of them not IV drug users, Haitians, or hemophiliacs. Six percent of all AIDS cases are now occurring in what—in insulting James Watt-ese—is called "the general population," i.e., people who are not gay, Haitian, hemophiliacs, or IV drug users.)

I return to find five letters on my desk. One announces a memorial service for my thirty-first friend who has died. The four others are from leading doctors involved with the AIDS epidemic. Each conveys the same message: Each doctor is frightened that the community is returning to the sexual freedoms of pre-AIDS days and that there is no visible gay political leadership in New York City to fight with the mayor and the Department of Health to force them to treat this epidemic with the same responsibility they would if it was happening in any other community. One letter, from the leading oncologist treating AIDS patients in New York, begs me to implore GMHC to plead with the gay community to observe complete sexual celibacy until the epidemic is stemmed.

I return to find that, after a few weeks of miraculously responsible journalism, *The New York Times* has regressed to its former silence on the subject of AIDS, while a raging epidemic is decimating its city. Until the day I die, I will never forgive this newspaper and this mayor for treating this epidemic, which is killing so many of my friends, in such an irresponsible fashion. This newspaper, which purports to record what is going on here to a population that includes one million gay people, has yet to do one human interest story on AIDS, to profile one patient, to do an in-depth article on GMHC, which represents one of the most amazing grass-roots responses by a community to taking care of its own. Day after day I see articles on every other charity and community and sufferer you can imagine. Never is there anything that deals with the human side of AIDS. (Or, for that matter, the human side of anything gay: Have you read much in the *Times* on SAGE, on Lambda, on any gay person beside Harvey Fierstein?) To *The New York Times*, we are still freaks, the homosexuals. Compare this to the *Washington Post*, which runs three to four sympathetic and moving articles every week. (Washington has thirty-two cases of AIDS.) Or the *Philadelphia Inquirer*, which, with the *Los Angeles Times*, leads the nation for the quality of its AIDS coverage. (Philadelphia has thirty-six cases.) No, I will never forgive *The New York Times*, late to arrive and early to leave. And by not maintaining their reporting on this crisis, they have helped to nurture our community into this false sense of security. (To see, day after day, their page after page of ads featuring gay-designed fashions is as morally repugnant as if Hebrew National had advertised in Hitler's favorite newspaper.)

It is no secret that I consider Mayor Koch to be, along with the *Times*, the biggest enemy gay men and women have to contend with in New York. Why does our gay leadership always act as if they are frightened of him? The sum total of this city's contributions to the AIDS epidemic to date is $24,500. That's it. Along with two meetings a month thrown in by a Department of Health that gives new meaning to the word "lethargy." Is it any wonder that in my Gay Pride Day speech I called Mayor Koch "a heartless, selfish son of a bitch?"

San Francisco's mayor, in a city that has 284 AIDS victims, has given $4 million to the organizations that provide to her city what GMHC provides for this one, including free buildings for patient services and money to remodel them. GMHC has been without a home for the two years of its existence, waiting, waiting, for the space the mayor's office promised over a year ago. When GMHC asked to use an abandoned and derelict high school on West 13th Street, the mayor demanded $2 million for it, cash up front, no terms, immediately. It would require an additional $800,000 to make it habitable. GMHC does not have this money, and in any event it considers it immoral to use donations received for patient care to pay the city for real estate the city should be providing free and would be providing free to any other community that was enduring an epidemic of death.

Because GMHC refuses to take advantage of the mayor's generous offer, it is being accused by other gay organizations of not being "community minded." Thus the mayor has succeeded in turning us against each other.

But GMHC must find larger quarters now. It has waited and waited until its activities can no longer be contained in the five tiny cubbyholes of a rooming house generously donated to it by two loyal members.

From here, over four hundred patients are supervised by over three hundred trained clinical volunteers each and every day. From here, over 1,500 Hotline phone calls are logged every week. From here, over 2 million pieces of printed literature giving the most up-to-date information have been dispatched all over the world. From here, twenty training sessions for doctors and nurses and Open Forums for the entire state are arranged each month.

And into these offices every week arrive ten new AIDS victims, seeking help. For them, GMHC provides crisis counseling, group therapy, welfare guidance, recreational activities, and hospital and home care. The demand for crisis counseling itself

is now so great that fifty new counselors must be trained each
month to join the 160 men and women who each look after one
or more patients—many of them, now, not gay—on a daily
basis. This counseling is the only loving contact most of these
victims ever receive.

To these tiny rooms come, each day, one hundred requests
for some sort of GMHC service. I have never seen a more
inspirational organization in operation anywhere in my life. I
have never witnessed a more fiscally responsible organization
in my life (certainly not in the gay community), and I have never
seen an organization catering to an epidemic that is the worst
in modern history treated so shabbily by a mayor, by a city, by
a federal government—or taken so much for granted by the
community it is trying to help.

GMHC comprises five hundred extremely active volunteers. There is a full-time staff of nine, two-thirds of whose
salaries are paid for by state grants. Less than one-third of
GMHC's budget is spent on administration. GMHC has raised
over $500,000 from benefits and small-donor contributions. It
has given away some $80,000 to local research that would oth-
erwise have been stopped, $12,000 to the National Gay Task
Force to help fund its own AIDS Hotline, $40,000 to help pay
a Washington lobbyist to fight for AIDS attention, and
$25,000 to the gay Community Health Project to continue its
vital AIDS screening program and diagnostic testing. That
this latter project is not being funded by the city or by the
Department of Health is shocking and offensive.

How dare Mayor Koch deny these committed and passion-
ate GMHC workers, desperately trying to care for an entire
epidemic virtually by themselves, the necessary space and
funding he would be providing to any other community—Jewish or Black or Poor or "General Population"—were AIDS happening to them?

And how dare the gay community not support the GMHC
Rodeo in Madison Square Garden on October 1st? Where else
is GMHC meant to find its money for all of these exhausting
services if not from us?

I appeal to the moral sense of obligation, to the sense of
what is right and must be done, of every gay person in this city

to come to GMHC's Rodeo at Madison Square Garden on October 1st. AIDS is not going to go away. Its cause is still invisible and its cure is still unfound. Treatment trials on every front are not very hopeful or promising. By the failure of gay men and lesbians to pack Madison Square Garden on October 1st, a message goes out to our mayor that our vote is not important, that he can continue to ignore us and our health crisis, and to our President and Congress and the world that their support is not necessary, and to AIDS victims that their care and cure is no longer on our minds.

We are asking the world to help us, to give us huge amounts of money to investigate this scourge. If we cannot help ourselves, we do not deserve anyone else's help.

Let's make another miracle. We have four days to sell ten thousand tickets.

This was published as an ad in the *Voice,* paid for (it cost $4,000) anonymously at the time by Joe Paschek, GMHC's treasurer, and his lover and business partner Lee Hulko. Joe was the financial genius who, from the very beginning, gave GMHC the impeccable and responsible fiscal security it still has; even though he was unhappy with me, he recognized the need for this ad.

I wrote it at the request of Rodger McFarlane, who was now GMHC's first full-time, paid executive director. Rodger inherited the Rodeo, which was probably a bad idea—to attempt to so quickly repeat the Circus success—and he saw an empty, yawning Madison Square Garden threatening only days before the event. It was not well attended, but somehow it managed to make a $75,000 profit. Most of the tickets were sold at the last minute.

I had returned not only from Europe but from Cape Cod, where I had written the first draft of *The Normal*

Heart, and I was on my way south, to an isolated log
cabin in Little Washington, Virginia, loaned me by old
friends, to write the second draft.

Because of my closeness to Rodger (we were then
living together as lovers as well), I felt I still had at least
some closeness to GMHC. Anyway, I continued to fight
for it publicly as loudly as I could. Rodger's relationship
with me, however, presented him with unnecessary
problems: Because of it, he was unable ever to truly win
the confidence of the Board, particularly of Paul Popham. Although he worked his ass off, and was responsible for running GMHC, magnificently, during the period
of its biggest growth (1983–85), the Board, now increased to include several more who also viewed me
unkindly, looked sceptically upon his total loyalty and
trustworthiness.

Paul became so distrustful of Rodger that at one
point he asked for a Board evaluation of his work. The
Board came back with the studied information that
Rodger was doing the work of ten people, and Paul had
egg all over his face. (When, in early 1985, *The Normal
Heart* opened, Rodger contributed a fact sheet on the
current status of the epidemic to be included with the
program; Paul was so furious at what he considered this
gesture of support of me that he recommended Rodger
be fired.)

During the next year and a half I was fully occupied
in rewriting my play and somehow finding a way to get
it produced. It was turned down by some fourteen play
agents. It was turned down by any number of directors
and producers and New York City and regional theatre
companies. It was turned down by American Playhouse
and PBS. But, with the help of Emmett Foster, who was
(and still is) personal assistant to Joseph Papp, and who
was also a GMHC volunteer, I was able to bring it to the
attention of this man who was to become so important
in my professional life.

Equal to Murderers

11 June 84

To:

Mr. Abe Rosenthal, *The New York Times*
Dr. Lawrence Altman, *The New York Times*
Mr. Tom Morgan, *The New York Times*
Judge Richard Failla, Gay Men's Health Crisis
Mr. Rodger McFarlane, Gay Men's Health Crisis
Mr. Paul Popham, Gay Men's Health Crisis
Ms. Virginia Apuzzo, National Gay Task Force
Dr. David Sencer, Commissioner of Health
Dr. Roger Enlow, Office of Gay and Lesbian Health
Mayor Edward Koch

    I am attaching an article from last Friday's *Washington Post* entitled "AIDS Epidemic Is Expanding, Not Shrinking, Experts Say." As you can see, this was a main, featured article, appearing on page A-3. It was sent to me by Tim Westmoreland, counsel to Representative Henry Waxman, who is Chair-

---

* *New York Native*, Issue 95, July 30–August 12, 1984.

man of the House Subcommittee on Health. Tim, like me, cannot understand why there is so little information passed on to the New York community about the appalling continuation, the march of this epidemic. After all, New York is still the worst hit. There are now *over four* new cases every day in this area, but you would not know it from reading *The New York Times*, or any of the literature put out by the above offices. The worst epidemic known to modern man is happening right here in this very city, and it is one of the best-kept secrets around.

All that is asked for, from all of you, is to transmit information, to keep an endangered population informed. Why is that so difficult?

That all of you listed above continue to refuse to transmit to the public the facts and figures of what is happening *daily* makes you, in my mind, equal to murderers, with blood on your hands just as if you had used knives or bullets or poison. Because you continue to refuse to inform New York's population, the perception by the average gay man on the street is that this epidemic has disappeared or leveled off or improved. Because of false hope (owing to the announcement that a virus has been isolated) that a cure will come tomorrow, the average gay man is back to living with his head in the sand. Because *The New York Times* is not reporting this vital news, because the city's Department of Health is not disseminating these appalling statistics, because the gay community's own organizations are too cowardly to speak out and speak up—all of this perpetuates the widespread ignorance that can only make for continued contagion, infection, and—at the present rate of increase—a minimum of 64,000 cases in two years' time.

In the name of God, Christ, Moses, whatever impels you to, at last, perform acts of humanity, when will you address this issue with the courage it demands?

During this week in June, gay health organizations sponsored a conference of several days, held at New

York University, to discuss many issues pertaining to the health, both mental and physical, of gay men and lesbians, and, only tangentially, AIDS.

By now Rodger and I had split up. I had failed in all three of my attempts to get back on GMHC's Board. I'd fought with Paul again, and again we no longer spoke. I was taking out my anger on Rodger for not supporting me—even if it meant he had to threaten to quit unless I was reinstated (a tactic that had certainly failed when I tried it).

I was appalled that so little of the health conference was devoted not only to AIDS but to any discussion of political action. After all we were continuing to endure, still no one was going after our enemies. GMHC by now was completely entrenched as a purely service agency, which angered me to the point of irrationality. Why couldn't they take stands? Why couldn't they advise men to cool it sexually?

I stood outside the conference entrance and handed out this letter to those attending. Then I went inside and interrupted the conference, yelling at them that they were not talking about what was *really* important. My reputation by now was completely that of a crazy man.

My use of the words "equal to murderers" in attacking my own people, my former lover, some of my former best friends, was not new. I had called them the same when I had been thrice rejected for re-admission to the Board. Yes, my reputation by now was completely that of a crazy man.

We Can Be Together

How to Organize the Gay Community

Here we are—another Gay Pride Day. We have a lot to be thankful for. We're still alive.

I have often been asked, "Okay, bigmouth, you're always yelling at us so much. Tell us what you think we should do. Be constructive."

So, at the risk of being yelled at even more, here is a list of Larry Kramer's suggestions: what we could be doing to get ourselves together for however many future years of gratitude we're going to be granted.

I

Organize. Okay, how do we organize? Well, you start with a few friends, and they get a few friends, and then you get all of them to get a few friends. You go from neighborhood to neighborhood, then from borough to borough, then from city to city, then from state to state, and then you've got the whole country. It is slow, thankless, necessary work, and until we do it—until we have one massive organization that represents *at least* one

* *Long Island Connection,* Vol. 4, Number 12, July 17, 1985.

million gay men and women—we'll still be victims of the system.

The biggest gay organizations in this country can only boast membership lists of 20,000 (GMHC) or 8,500 (NGTF). That's shocking. The National Rifle Association, Jerry Falwell's Moral Majority—they get what they want because they can prove they have mailing lists of millions of people. When they send out requests to these millions to write letters to Congress, those letters get written and responded to. That's how you get things in this country. That's how democracy works. Visible pressure from visible numbers. And there's not that much wrong with the idea. What's wrong is our inability to put this method into action ourselves.

Now we have a choice to make. Do we want to add our names to the lists of already existing organizations—GMHC, NGTF, Gay Rights National Lobby, all of which have very poor records of fighting for us, and all of which are controlled by boards of directors who are timid sissies, old ladies, old men, old farts, useless—or do we, somehow, try to start a brand-new organization from scratch?

I would dearly like to see the latter—something new is often better than something tired. But something new, to be effective, takes money, lots of money. I am talking about hundreds of thousands of dollars, maybe a million. It also takes a leader, and we have precious few of them. I would like to see such a new beginning, but until a gay Rockefeller comes along and plunks down the start-up funds, I don't see it happening. And we can't afford to do it on the cheap again—that's the trouble with NGTF and GRNL: They haven't got the funds to stay in shape; they're in debt; and it's hard to do good work when you're in debt.

Therefore, for the present, we don't have much choice but to try to make our existing organizations better. Pump some blood and energy into those sagging, wheezing carcasses. How can we do this? Well, believe it or not, we accomplish this by joining them. We get in touch with GMHC, with NGTF, with GRNL, and we say to them: I will join your organization; here is my contribution. *But*—and this is the biggest of big *buts*—I am giving you this money and at the same time I am telling you I don't think you are doing a good enough job. I am giving you this money to *fight*. To establish as powerful a lobbying presence in Washington as you can. We simply must have our own people fighting for us in Washington, and you are not doing that. In taking my twenty-five dollars (or whatever it is) you must pledge to me that this money will be used for political fighting and only that. At a recent East End Gay Organization meeting, I was thrilled to hear my remarks met with a pledge by their president that they would try to raise, among themselves, part or all of the amount it costs to maintain one lobbyist in Washington—$60,000.

This gives rise to another possibility. That you and your friends could start fund-raising on your own to pay for a lobbyist's salary. If groups and organizations all over this country would each commit themselves to raising $60,000 a year, we would have a platoon of lobbyists in Washington that would be impressive. Don't worry about finding the right person. We have contacts in Washington that can locate him or her.

To give you an example of why lobbyists in Washington are our first priority, let me cite what not having them has meant. "The" AIDS virus was isolated in France fifteen months before Washington announced that our scientists had "discovered" it. The Centers for Disease Control in Atlanta wanted to put this French virus to work immediately, in those vital tests that will help us make progress toward a cure, a vaccine, and blood tests. But they were told, "Don't you dare use the French virus. We, the government, have poured millions of dollars into our own research; you wait until we discover our own virus." I put this simplistically, of course, but that's the essence. For fifteen months a virus had been isolated that could have helped research move ahead. If we had had lobbying power in Washington, we could have charged in and said: "No, sir, you use that French virus immediately, or I tell my membership of one million (2 million, 3 million) about the hanky-panky that's going on and some of you might not get reelected." (Why didn't GMHC fight for the use of the French virus?)

Did you know that the majority of the funds allocated to AIDS research goes not to finding a cure, but to finding a vaccine, producing blood tests—to almost anything but to improve the chances of the sick and dying? If we had people in Washington fighting for us, we could fight to right that imbalance. We could fight for our lives, which we must do now. Getting as many people as possible representing us in Washington—our people, paid for by us—is top priority. And our present organizations are not doing this, either fast enough or at all.

GMHC will give you the feeble excuse that it is a not-for-profit organization and is thus prohibited by law from participating in political action. You don't think the Catholic Church, the Salvation Army, the American Cancer Society haven't found ways to become political without losing their not-for-profit status? An organization is prohibited from spending *over a certain percentage* of its income on political activity. It doesn't take any money to have a troop of volunteers sit down and write letters—the cheapest, most effective way of making your voice heard. It doesn't cost any money to have a troop of volunteers picket City Hall for their inattention to the AIDS crisis. It doesn't cost any money to have a troop of volunteers flood switchboards with complaints when *The New York Times* runs something ignorant and hateful.

Ironically, appallingly, when you come to GMHC to offer your services as a volunteer, they will tell you, "We don't need any volunteers right now—we're all filled up." Can you imagine an organization with as much to do as it has, refusing the services of volunteers? That path only leads to stagnation and death. You must say to them: "I think this is the stupidest thing I have ever heard—but write down my name and phone number anyway, and when you are ready to form a political-action division, please call me." And when you haven't heard from them after a week or two, call them back and say: "I am still waiting to volunteer my services for a political-action division." After a while, they will get the message.

It is possible for you to let those foul boards of directors of GMHC, or NGTF, or GRNL know that they are all sitting on their hands. Simply call each organization directly and say you would like to have a list of their board members and their addresses. They are obligated to send such a list to you. Then write to each director and say: "If you don't care enough to fight harder, do you think you could relinquish your seat to someone who will and can?"

II

Organize. Okay, so now you have sent your membership donations to GMHC, to GRNL, to NGTF, and you have got a group of twenty-five of your friends to join with a group of twenty-five of somebody else's friends and the fifty of you are thinking about joining with another fifty that has similarly organized in Brooklyn. How do you keep the damn thing from falling apart? What's your agenda? How do you keep everyone active and busy and interested and committed—before they get bored out of their minds and return to the baths and drugs? How do you sustain energy?

My answer to that is that every one of us—women, too—must repeat to ourselves, like a catechism, over and over: *Each and every minute of my life, I must act as if I already have AIDS and am fighting for my life.*

It also means that each of the one hundred members that you now have can and should work at least one night a week at one of these organizations. (There is no local office of GRNL, but that does not mean there couldn't be.) When you work as a volunteer for an organization, get to know the other volunteers, the staff, and the board members. (Board members rarely show up at their organizations; some of them don't even know what their organizations do. But you're going to change all that.) Get to know the lay of the land. And as you do, let them get to know you and why you're there and what you stand for. *You stand for fighting.* Fighting to get lobbying power in Washington. Fighting to get Mayor Koch to do something, anything, for AIDS. Fighting to get *The New York Times* and every magazine and publication you read or come across to pay more attention to the tragedies that we as gay people face all the time but see so little written about: AIDS, immigration, discrimination in jobs and housing, the nerve of Archbishop— pardon me, Cardinal—O'Connor. There are many, many issues.

In fact, now that you have your own little organization going, one order of business could be each of you, there on the spot, sitting down and writing a letter to the same person. One hundred letters sent at one time to *The New York Times,* to Mayor Koch, to Senator D'Amato, are going to be seen and read. If they don't respond, write them again.

Establish goals. This can mean tracking down the person or persons you think responsible for some fault, or the person or persons you think might be able to help you do something about it. If a friend of yours who has AIDS has been treated badly in a hospital, find out who at that hospital can help you to see that it won't happen again. If you want to know what Senator Moynihan's or Senator D'Amato's position is on AIDS and how much they have done about it (next to nothing), locate someone working for them, both here in New York and in Washington, and establish a relationship on the phone with that person. You will find out that one phone call will lead to another—and, good detective that you are, you will pursue your goal like the best of bloodhounds. You will be paid attention to if you say "I represent the Long Island Chapter of Gay———; we have one hundred members in our chapter and we are affiliated with other chapters that bring our total membership to over one thousand, and we feel that you are not doing enough to fight for us."

Constantly keep your goals in view. Constantly reassess your goals, and your progress in reaching them. Be realistic, but also challenge yourself to try to do more and more, reach further, fight harder. Constantly remind yourself of what it's all about.

So now you have an organization going that has one hundred members and each of you also spends one night a week or one hour a week volunteering for GMHC or NGTF or some other gay organization that you are interested in putting into fighting shape, and each of you is also writing one letter a week to protest one of the many indignities we endure every day. Where do you go from here? Are you so tired now that you are fed up and disgusted, and have returned to your former state of Doing Nothing About It? *Just remember the old battle cry: Each and every minute of my life, I must act as if I already have AIDS and am fighting for my life.*

If this continues to give you energy, and I pray to heaven that it does, now you must try to connect your organization with another organization that has been growing in membership, too. This is called networking, and historically gay organizations have been terrible at it. We've simply never been able to get along, particularly in New York, the most competitive and brutal of cities. But once again, we simply have to grit our teeth, repeat our catechism, and try. It's do-or-die time, fellas and girls.

The most convenient way of networking locally is right under our noses. At present, it's a mess. But it's there, in place, and ready for rehabilitation. Once a month there meets a very peculiar organization. It is called the Community Council, and ostensibly it is composed of one representative from every existing organization in New York that has asked to join and has paid its dues. In its heyday, there must have been sixty or seventy constituent members. Now I understand there are less than a dozen. This is a pity. The Community Council is potentially a very good starting point for getting us some power in New York City. It really should be put back into shape—with reconstituted goals. Just think of how many gay organizations there are: GMHC, NGTF, Men of All Colors Together, the various choruses and music groups, Salsa Soul Sisters, the political clubs, gay alumni groups from Yale and elsewhere. These are groups with combined memberships that must approach at least fifty thousand. If every gay organization in the area got themselves back onto the Community Council, I think we could start something rolling.

In the past, this organization had no power, because it had no elected officers and chose not to take any strong stands. It was a monthly forum for screaming. Meetings of the full Community Council were, quite frankly, revolting. Nobody would listen to anybody else. To get a consensus on anything—even the time—was next to impossible.

So why am I offering up this den of vipers as something filled with hope and potential? Because it is there, it is in place. What is not in place is machinery to make the Community Council effective. It must change its modus operandi. It must elect officers, it must take political stands on all issues, and it must make these stands heard. It must organize, just as you have done.

That the Mayor of New York has ignored us for so long is something the new Community Council can take a stand on. You let City Hall know that the mayor is expected to march in our parade. It is appalling that he has refused to do so for so long. That Mayor Koch refused to give us, for free, a falling-down building for our community center is shocking. The Community Council, if it had teeth, could have demanded that we be *given* that building, for which we paid $1.5 million. It's still not too late. That Mayor Koch has continually assigned us a useless liaison to the gay community is equally unacceptable. First we had the hated Herb Rickman. Well, we did manage to get rid of him. Now we have sweet Lee Hudson, who is, I'm afraid, only a figurehead. She can't *do* anything. Who can blame her if she has trouble defending Koch's position on almost any gay issue you can think of? At a recent meeting, she put forth Koch's Office of Gay and Lesbian Health Concerns as a positive step that Koch has taken for our community. I said, "Indeed it was—but then why did he keep it without a head for almost a year?"

A strong Community Council could have a lot to say about who gets that job. And about seeing that the Office of Gay and Lesbian Health Concerns *does* something.

Ed Koch knows he is in trouble with the gay community. He was booed at the AIDS benefit at the Shubert Theatre. I consider him to be the one person most responsible for letting the AIDS epidemic get out of hand. He is now going around trying to "make nice" to us. He appeared at the gay synagogue, made a little speech, and answered questions. (It has taken him five years to accept their invitation.) This is the man who, in five years, has given a total of $75,000 to community AIDS services, compared with San Francisco's $16 million. A strong Community Council, with you and your group a part of it, could roundly and loudly protest this inhumanity.

If you have AIDS in San Francisco, you are eligible to enter one of the best hospital wards in this country—the AIDS section of San Francisco General Hospital. Visit a few AIDS patients in almost any hospital in New York, and you are liable to hear stories that make your hair stand on end. If you get AIDS in San Francisco, you are eligible for a whole assortment of services that you cannot get in New York—housing, crisis counseling of a kind that GMHC is no longer able to offer, a faster and more responsive welfare system. You don't get any of these things without fighting for them. Why hasn't GMHC fought Mayor Koch harder for these things? Why haven't we made GMHC fight harder? You could come down with AIDS tomorrow. Do you want to be treated like a San Francisco gay or a New York gay? *Each and every minute of my life, I must act like I already have AIDS and am fighting for my life.*

III

Organize. Now that you are on the Community Council, and it has been turned into a responsive, responsible organization, it is time to turn toward national objectives. You must locate the equivalent of the Community Council in every town and city that you can. And representatives must meet regularly to cement ideas on how to network area by area, region by region, across the country.

It is through this kind of network that we could plan a march on Washington and make it work. I am here to tell you that if one million gay people marched on Washington, they would see us and hear us. I am not talking about 10,000 or 100,000. These numbers march in Washington every other weekend. Political power comes from *numbers,* and numbers mean *visibility,* and optimum visibility is a march on Washington of one million women and men. Oh, Mother of God, would that not be a day of Glory! Hallelujah! Why is it such a dream? Why couldn't we bring it off? With you and your friends and their friends, it just might happen. And once we have marched on Washington, we must do it again. And again. And again. Like anti-war protestors did against our country's involvement in Vietnam.

I have for some time been putting forth the notion of a Summit Meeting. What I have in mind is that leaders from all over America would come to a central place and sit in a room and say, "Okay, for this meeting we are all going to get along together and work out some way to organize our national gay community into a working mechanism that can become a presence in Washington." Such a Summit Meeting would be fraught with every problem imaginable—people in groups have a hard time agreeing on anything. But I cling to the hope that with the threat of AIDS we might just be able to put on our crisis wardrobe and get on with it at last.

It is through a national organization that we could achieve most. Our very own organization, powerful, strong, with a huge mailing list, in Washington, on the spot, just like the

National Rifle Association, the Moral Majority, the American Red Cross, General Motors. Everyone who is anything has an office in Washington. And we don't. Some 24 million gay men and lesbians have no office in Washington. How ludicrous a situation. What a death wish.

An office in Washington, a building in Washington, a troop of lobbyists in Washington—these mean something. Just as *not* having any of these means something. Without them we are prepared to die, and without a whimper of protest. A recent issue of a powerful Washington newsletter, read on Capitol Hill, had a lead article that said, in essence: "You, the senators and representatives and power brokers who are reading this, don't have to worry about the gay vote, about the gay community, because they are unorganized, because they have no representatives in Washington, because they are powerless. Therefore you don't have to vote for anything pro-gay, and if you vote anti-gay, don't worry about it—they won't even know it or fight back." Many senators and representatives and lobbyists read this. Please God, may that scare the shit out of you and get you off your ass and into action.

I cannot overestimate the necessity of this desperately needed political presence in Washington.

IV

Organize. Here are two other things to think about:

Help force Ed Koch and Carol Bellamy into helping us. We are about to have a mayoral race between a "confirmed bachelor" and an "unmarried woman." Because both of them are so terrified of being perceived as gay, they bend over backwards to ignore us. They are going to be making a lot of campaign promises now. We must make Koch promise us everything he has denied us. If either of them wants the gay vote, they must be honest about gay issues. *Whoever opens the closet first gets my vote.*

We are fortunate in this area to have two gay newspapers that get better with every issue, the *Long Island Connection* and the *New York Native*. [The *Connection* ceased publication shortly after this appeared.] Make sure you and your friends read these papers. This is the best way I know of keeping up to date on what is happening about AIDS. If every gay man and lesbian reads them, these papers make a little more money, which means they can afford to extend their coverage. You might even write to Bloomingdale's or some other favorite store and ask them: "Why aren't you advertising in the gay press? I buy from you—why don't you support my papers?"

But other gay newspapers are not so good, and they should be told they are not so good. The *Advocate*, this country's leading gay newspaper in terms of sales, has its priorities in the wrong place, has had its head in the sand for too long. The *Advocate* lives in the Age Before AIDS. The mentality of this newspaper is strictly laid-back California est, Hawaiian shirts, and guest houses in Key West. Every article sounds as if it was written by the same person who engages in no serious discussions of anything controversial. You might write a few letters to the *Advocate* as long as you're writing.

The *Washington Blade*, as our presence in Washington, is equally as shocking in its lack of zeal, its reluctance to crusade in a city where it could do the most good. The *New York Native* has a woman in Washington, Ann Fettner, writing some of the best AIDS pieces around. How is it that the *Connection* can in one issue present more political news than the *Blade* can present in several months? Why can't we have a dynamic, fighting newspaper in our capital, exerting pressure where it's needed most? Another great opportunity tragically wasted.

How are we to know what is going on if we do not have an effective network of newspapers? If *The New York Times* and the *Chicago Tribune* and the *L.A. Times* aren't going to write about us, and if the *Advocate* and the *Blade* lack the interest or resolve to crusade, if the gay papers in almost every city other than New York fall far short of what we need, how are we going to get the word out—about anything?

The *San Francisco Chronicle* is blessed with an openly gay reporter, Randy Shilts. In the first ten months of 1984, the *Chronicle* ran 163 articles about AIDS. God bless you, Randy. Compare this with the puny, paltry numbers of thirty-seven in the L.A. *Times*, and twenty-four in the *Washington Post*. Why doesn't the *Advocate* raise a stink about this in its California pages? Why doesn't the *Blade* raise a stink about this in its

Washington pages? *Each and every minute of my life, I must act as if I already have AIDS and am fighting for my life.*

Okay, here comes the hardest question of all. How are we all going to get along with each other in order to get any of this done? I certainly include myself here. I have a bad temper; I am impatient with anybody who doesn't agree with me—and all of you are probably a bit of the same. I have no real answers to this. I have already fucked up once, woefully, in my relationship with GMHC. If we could only sit down together in the same room (which GMHC will not do with me), saying and thinking our catechism, putting up a few pictures in our mind's eye of our friends who have died, maybe we might be able to do it.

We gays are still as children in this political game. We are inexperienced. But day by day and month by month we learn a little more. And in learning we acquire skills. Perhaps, touched by political reality, after we've bitched each other to death, we will learn how to negotiate, how to compromise, how to give a little. I know I have said, "I will never forgive the Board of GMHC," and "I will never forgive Mayor Koch." But GMHC and I are both different entities now from what we were when we commenced our quarrels three years ago. Doesn't it make more sense to have your critics on your side? It seems to me the secret of a successful organization is the ability to accommodate all views—not closing out those in opposition. This, after all, is the secret of America. (GMHC has shut out all opposing voices—and they have systematically made certain that access to the organization was and is denied to anyone who does not think as they do. Ask me, ask Dr. Joseph Sonnabend, ask Michael Callen, ask Jim Fouratt.) If GMHC is to regain strength, if NGTF, GRNL, the Community Council, *all of us*, are to find new strength, it can only be in one room, together. Just as political enemies face each other daily in Congress. Being gay people, what if we tried to hug each other, even a little? (Imagine Koch and Kramer hugging. Well, stranger things have happened.)

Togetherness is numbers. Togetherness is unity. Unity is strength. Strength is power. Power is acceptance. Acceptance is a certain kind of Equality.

Let me say a few final words about leadership. Over the

years, we have had precious few leaders who stayed around long enough to achieve anything. It seems that no sooner does a good one come along than he or she has some hidden agenda: to use his or her gay leadership position to get a better-paying political job, for instance.

In most cases, however, the quality of our leadership has been second-rate. Good people do not want to get involved in gay politics—and who can blame them? It is, as I started this article by noting, a thankless job. But now is a time for sacrifice. These are the years of death and dying, the plague years, and they are here to stay.

So we must obey certain moral imperatives, commandments if you will, just as if we were devout practitioners of any religion that calls for service, for giving. We must give to the cause of Gay Rights all that we have to give. We must urge, beg, implore every potential leader we know to become actively involved. We know who among our friends is better able than others: who has valuable skills—for reasoning, for public speaking, for common sense, for passion. Or who has money. God, how money is needed. We know whom among us we respect, to whom we listen, to whom we go when we need advice. These are our potential leaders: your lawyer, your accountant, your professors, your doctors. Tell them they must devote their brains and skills and passions to helping make us stronger *politically*.

It is from among these people that we will find our leaders, our fighters. Many of them are still in the closet at work, perhaps even at home. We must implore them to hide no longer. It is up to each one of us to pass along this message: No longer will any excuse be tolerated for shying away from responsibility. Not if these people wish to continue enjoying our respect. Yes. Shame them into participation, if necessary. We simply must field a better qualified set of leaders to represent us in the coming years. We need them locally (New York has the most poorly organized gay community of any major city); we need them in Washington; we need them everywhere.

So help locate these men and women. Ask them to join your own group of twenty-five or fifty. Tell them to bring their colleagues, those they respect and admire. Make your group as tough and smart and agile as you can. Let us field our best fighting power—and we will be respected adversaries in due course.

All of this, I know, sounds exhausting. But which of us does not have a few spare hours a week? Or an evening? Which of us does not have a few hundred dollars? Or a piece of paper and a pen? Or a telephone?

And who among us does not have friends? Friends to join our first small organization?

Who among us does not know a potential leader—a doctor, a lawyer, a scientist, someone from Harvard or NYU? I do not mean to sound elitist, but with education comes responsibility, and if ever we needed responsible, well-educated, presentable leaders, it is now.

Every single one of us can and must answer all the above questions with "That's me. I do."

For every single one of us faces the possibility that he might be dead, very shortly, in a few years, perhaps in a few months.

Did you know that scientists and doctors are now thinking that the AIDS virus may have been around for as long as *twenty* years? That someone you fucked with twenty years ago could have transmitted the virus to you? So that even if you have lived in a monogamous relationship for nineteen years, you still might not be completely in the clear. We're all walking time bombs, waiting for whatever it is to set us off.

Each and every minute of my life, I must act as if I already have AIDS and am fighting for my life.

I devoted 1985 and 1986 mostly to *The Normal Heart*. I finally had a hit show. During and after the almost-year-long run at Joe Papp's Public Theater in New York, where it starred first Brad Davis and then Joel Grey, there were productions in Los Angeles (with Richard Dreyfuss), at the Long Wharf in New Haven (with Tom Hulce), at the Royal Court in London (with Martin Sheen), transferring to the West End (Tom Hulce again,

and then John Shea), and, after these, at just about
every major regional theatre in America and by companies around the world, including such unlikely places as
Poland, where a production was so successful that it's
being repeated on Polish television. Poland is a country
where homosexuality is so frowned upon that gay suicides are common. I rarely allow myself to feel good
about having written something that might help change
people's minds. I never think that happens. But it was
nice to have a success.

Some two years of negotiations with Barbra Streisand for the film rights (she was to produce, direct, and
play the part of Dr. Emma Brookner) came to nothing
but $20,000 in legal fees for me. People predicted from
the start we were two impossibly difficult people who
could never come to terms. When she first called me, she
was filled with excitement and passion, both for my play
and the problems it dramatizes. Her own agent, Stan
Kamen of William Morris, with whom I'd been told she
was exceptionally close, had just died from AIDS. I was
interested in her filming it mainly because I figured she
would draw a larger world audience to the film than
anyone I could think of. But I was soon forced into
realizing that her excitement and passion were an up
and down thing. It was not until I met her, some many
months after negotiations began (it takes a very long
time to deal with someone with so many lawyers, man-
agers, agents, partners, assistants, secretaries, and personal attendants) that she had decided to make another
film first, which I'd not been told originally. And this
film, *Nuts*, was one that not only suffered delay after
delay, but was awful when it finally came out, by which
time I no longer wanted her to film *The Normal Heart*.

But, for these two years, she had me in a bind:
Negotiations dragged on and on, never fully completed,
so I was not free to go elsewhere without fear of her
legal reprisals. In essence, she not only sat on me and
my play, but effectively saw to it that no one else could
bring this subject to the screen—an action that I think

was selfish and exceedingly inhumane. While I enjoyed my creative meetings with her (she is a very smart woman), she would not agree to guarantee that I would be the only screenwriter. I gave in on this point, and hated myself (and by extension, her) for doing so.

For a while, I toyed with the idea of directing the film myself. Many of the stars who had played Ned Weeks were willing to allow me to direct them, and the magnificent Linda Hunt agreed to play my Emma. But money was not so available for this novice director as I'd hoped, even with such a fine cast as I was able to assemble, and even with my old friend Paul Maslansky (who'd done so well with his many *Police Academies*) as the producer.

Just when the matter of a film appeared to be dead, another old friend, and former boss, David Picker (who, as head of United Artists, had been responsible for allowing me to script *Women in Love*), appeared once again in his role of White Knight. He is now setting up the film, and if all goes well, we may just make it to the screen at last.

By now I'd learned that no matter what I wrote and said and did, I was going to get flak from somewhere. But for the first time in my writing career, there wasn't much criticism against *The Normal Heart*. What little there was came from gay critics who accused me of writing "a self-serving revenge play" against the Board of GMHC, making myself the hero. I'm sorry they saw the play so narrowly. I tried to make Ned Weeks as obnoxious as I could. He isn't my idea of a hero. He fucks up totally. He yells at his dying lover and screams and rants and raves at and against everyone and everything else and gets tossed out of "the organization" on his ass. I was trying, somehow and again, to atone for my own behavior. I tried to make Bruce Niles, the Paul Popham character, the sympathetic leader he in fact was. I hoped Paul would come and see the play, which he would not do, and be honored.

But I also wanted to show that these were our fights that kept us diminished and divided. I think they're fights not dissimilar to those in any growing organization, gay or straight, and that they probably can't be avoided, or afforded.

One peculiar fallout from the play, and from my other political writing, is my being pegged as an advocate of celibacy. I don't think I've ever advocated that, or urged anything but caution, and "cooling it." Characters in *The Normal Heart* may have said other things (as they did and do in real life), but it's a selfish and vicious critic who can so yank a line or two of dialogue out of context to nail the author with it as his sworn message. I was against promiscuity long before *The Normal Heart;* I believe being gay offers much more than that. But proponents (even in this age of AIDS) of promiscuity—which is far different from sexual freedom, which I, of course, support—have made me their enemy. I do confess to not knowing where one draws the line between caution and disregard. That is everyone's personal decision to make when he or she is completely informed of all that is known. But I am not so dumb as to believe that an entire population can stop having sex. Nor do I think it's healthy for many that they do so.

After the main productions, I found it increasingly difficult to sit through the play any more. It contains too many unhappy memories. (It also contains too much clumsy writing.) I wrote it to make people cry: AIDS is the saddest thing I'll ever have to know. I also wrote it to be a love story, in honor of a man I loved who died. I wanted people to see on a stage two men who loved each other. I wanted people to see them kiss. I wanted people to see that gay men in love and gay men suffering and gay men dying are just like everyone else.

Second-Rate Voice

How sad that the *Village Voice* would not publish Anna Mayo's excellent AIDS article ("The Principle of Uncertainty," *Native*, 151). How much sadder *Voice* editor Robert Friedman's excuse, as reported in the *Native*, for not doing so: "I felt the end product was too speculative. It didn't convince me." If we had to wait for convincing evidence on practically any aspect of AIDS, we would have nothing to read at all. No—the major important job every publication should be performing for its readers (and the one the *Native* has been accomplishing better than any other publication in the world) is to allow all theories to be aired, crackpot as they may seem—*now*. Last week I would have considered any radiation theory crackpot; last night I watched a "60 Minutes" segment on radiation contamination as the cause of leukemia in children in Wareham, Massachusetts.

I think I know as much about AIDS as any layperson. I do not fully believe anything I have read or seen or heard about. I am not a hundred percent convinced about any theory or set of "facts" about anything beyond the fact that our lives are

* *New York Native*, Issue 152, March 17, 1986.

filled with such an unfair and inhuman tragedy as to propagate madness—of all kinds. I think every single person, *without exception,* who is making *major* decisions about AIDS, for this country, for this state, for this city, for the mainstream media—is second-rate. They are second-rate scientists, second-rate doctors, second-rate epidemiologists, second-rate journalists, second-rate intelligences. There is not a first-rate brain among them.

Therefore I think it is imperative that all theories be aired, so we can each listen, sift, combine, question for ourselves, and make our own decisions. It is incumbent on the editor of each serious publication to provide space and outlet for serious speculation.

Over the past five and one-half years, I have become so disillusioned with the concept of our "free press" that I can now read Solzhenitsyn as a brother and not as a foreigner. If we have to "convince" Robert Friedman, Abe Rosenthal, Ben Bradlee, and Dan Rather that there is a story going on here as atrocious as any atrocity story the Second World War produced, then we are in trouble.

We are, of course, in trouble. We are in great trouble. Our troubles become greater and more perilous with each second. I do not need to call New Yorkers' attention to what appears to be yet another wave of new deaths and diagnoses among our friends. I do not have to call any perceptive gay person's attention to the fact that we are as politically unorganized, both locally and nationally, as we have ever been, that we are still in no way equipped to face the horrors that are coming down the pike. I do not have to tell anyone how tired we all are—physically, emotionally, spiritually—as individuals and as a community. Quite frankly, I despair.

It is imperative that we know that we have no friends to help us in many quarters where we think we have them. We have no friends at the Centers for Disease Control. We have no friends at the U.S. Department of Health and Human Services. We have no friends at the New York City Department of Health. We have fewer friends at an increasing number of New York City hospitals. (A very dear friend of mine was turned away by a doctor at New York Hospital when he had a suspected case of AIDS, with the statement, uttered quite openly and baldly, "I no longer take any gay patients." At New York Hospital!)

And, it saddens me to say, we have no friends at the *Village Voice*. We must not forget that this paper has, quite possibly, as bad a record on AIDS coverage as any paper in America. It was May 1983, a grotesque twenty-three months after the epidemic was officially declared, before they ran their first major article (by Stephen Harvey). During this agonizing period, gay writers constantly submitted ideas and requests, only to be treated badly. "They were obnoxious" is how one free-lance gay writer remembers his treatment. Many of us simply couldn't believe the *Voice* was doing this to us. We understood *The New York Times* not writing about us; that we were accustomed to. Dr. Lawrence Mass, the award-winning medical journalist to whom the gay community owes so much for his pioneering reporting on AIDS in the *Native*, was actually commissioned by the *Voice*, in November 1982, to write an AIDS piece. "The Most Important New Public Health Problem in the United States" was the title of the article he submitted. After three months of sitting on it, the *Voice* refused to run it. "It's not a *Voice* piece," was what senior editor Karen Durbin told Mass, in no way allowing him the opportunity to rework or resubmit the article. The *Native* ran it immediately.

Voice coverage to this day is spotty, second-rate, unimaginative, out-of-date, or stuff we have read earlier elsewhere. In Richard Goldstein, their openly gay senior editor, we have a first-rate example of the Uncle Toms among us—openly gay people who do nothing to help us, when they are in positions where they easily could. I would not like to live with Goldstein's conscience, all these years of being at the *Voice* and not writing or assigning AIDS articles when he should have been. How an openly gay senior editor could sit on his ass for the first twenty-three months of an epidemic that was, and still is, decimating his brothers, defies comprehension. Not that his record has been all that much better since. No, we must not forget the shameful silence of the *Voice*, as we must not forget the shameful silence of *The New York Times* for not writing about the Final Solution when it happened.

I was greatly encouraged when, last year, the *Voice* was purchased by Leonard Stern, the business partner of one of my closest friends. I was even more encouraged when someone I knew, Robert Friedman, was appointed the new editor. Both Leonard and Robert promised me that AIDS would immediately become top priority. At Robert's invitation, I submitted to him (and continue to do so) lists of possible AIDS stories and lists of good writers to write them. Alas, if anything, AIDS coverage at the *Voice* is even less than it was during the previous regime. The paper that takes such delight and relish in exposing every latest juicy tidbit about the Koch administration refuses to write about what history will prove to be the biggest scandal in the Koch administration—their heinous handling of the AIDS crisis from day one until this very day. (Dr. Mathilde Krim released the most damning report on what Koch has not done on AIDS; why did no New York newspaper other than the *Native* report on this? Isn't this the stuff the *Voice* I used to love and respect—many long years ago—would trumpet to the skies?)

For the life of me, I don't understand why this situation continues. Stern is not out to kill us. Friedman is not a monster. Even Goldstein, much as I detest what he stands for, can do good work. I think each would consider himself to be a caring person, devoted to at least some of the principles of humanism. And yet, week after week, all they turn out are more issues filled with pointless tripe, filled with pages and pages of critics with their jerk-off reviews, sounding off on what's on the tube, what's playing in the latest loft, where you can buy the trendiest spaghetti or eat it, who was seen at what stupid movie preview, what undiscovered rock song/star/ballet/mixed media simply must be discovered, what film director/playwright/novelist/poet/painter has a career that's too big and overinflated or too small and underappreciated. Have you ever seen a publication that devoted so much of its valuable space to so many saying so little you care about reading? While we are dying. While the "Village" part of the *Village Voice* is dying.

One of the saddest lessons I have learned from this epidemic is that the true heterosexual liberal, for some unaccountable reason, is not necessarily the gay person's friend. He or she will fight for blacks, women, Hispanics, abortion, nuclear disarmament, keeping the Jefferson Library open all week. But when it comes to homosexuality, they get queasy. Figure that one out. I can't.

Just as, for the life of me, I can't understand why the *Village Voice* is so stinking awful on gay issues in general and AIDS in particular. I can see no reason for any gay person to read this paper; in fact, I think we should avoid it at present.

An Open Letter to Richard Dunne and Gay Men's Health Crisis

Dear Richard,

The Doomsday Scenario that many have feared for so long comes closer. Next week, 274 people will die from AIDS. Next week, 374 more will become infected with the killer virus. In four years' time, 270,000 people will have AIDS. Of these, 179,000 will have died. Around the globe, many millions already are infected. As many as 50 percent of these millions will die.

Two out of three AIDS cases in America are still happening to gay men.

For all the worthy Patient Services and Education that have been provided, the rate of infection and death continues unabated.

As presently constituted, organized, and managed, Gay Men's Health Crisis, Inc., of which you are Executive Director, is simply not equipped or prepared or able to deal with an emergency of this magnitude.

This letter is an urgent plea to you and your Board of Directors to wake up, look coldly and harshly at the realities you have been ignoring for so long, and reconstitute yourselves so

* *New York Native*, Issue 197, January 26, 1987.

that at last you perform the actions you were established to perform in the first place: to fight for gay men—that we may go on living.

For the past five years I have painfully watched as GMHC has attempted to be all things to all people, in so doing losing complete sight of the larger picture, of what is happening, of what you should be doing and are not doing.

I call for nothing less than a total reassessment of your goals and a rethinking of what you are there for, what we need you there for, and what you must accomplish for us.

This letter has been in my mind for some time. I have not written it before because I kept hoping someone up there would come to his or her senses. This has not happened, and the action that finally prompted this letter is this:

In *The New York Times* of January 10th, you are quoted (concerning the release by ICN Pharmaceuticals of its most promising ribavirin data at a press conference) as follows: "We cannot understand why they chose to raise the hopes of so many people by releasing their clinical trial information through a press conference instead of a more responsible manner such as an appropriate medical journal."

I prayed that you did not say this. I prayed that the Executive Director of the organization that is meant to fight for the rights of gay men—men and rights that have been constantly, continuously denied, with a disregard for us bordering on the murderous—did not say this to a newspaper and to a world filled with heterosexual connivance, bordering on collusion at the least and conspiracy at the most—ignoring us, treating us like so much offal fit to die in agony while tests, trials, delays, ignorance, inhumane uncaring, lying, and ass-dragging characterize the daily activities of just about everyone and everything in sight, particularly the "appropriate medical journals."

I do not give a flying fuck what the *New England Journal of Medicine* reports about AIDS, or *Science* or *Lancet* or the *Journal of the American Medical Association*. From the very beginning of this epidemic they have shown scant humane concern for us, for our rights, for our continued healthy survival on this planet. Indeed, one of the main reasons this epidemic became an epidemic was that the *New England Journal of Medicine*—that "responsible . . . appropriate medical journal"—would not accept papers of warning from leading doctors observing a new phenomenon that they wished to warn the world about quickly, when they had little clinical data or test results, only observation. For an entire year, doctors at New York University and UCLA Medical Centers could not get the *New England Journal of Medicine*—that "responsible . . . appropriate medical journal"—to publish their frightening observations. And, of course, during that year, that crucial first year, an epidemic that could have been controlled and contained got woefully out of hand. These "responsible . . . appropriate medical journals" have scarcely been better since. How dare you be so trusting and naïve—you who are head of Gay Men's Health Crisis!

Why could you not applaud them? The ribavirin data *is* promising, as Dr. Mathilde Krim had the good sense to remark in the *Times*, "but not conclusive" (which no one is stating it is). From such encouragement can come swifter action at the FDA level, can come swifter and further tests, can come the release and availability of this drug to a wider market—can come all the things those who are dying so desperately pray for: PROGRESS.

But what does Auntie GMHC say and sound like? You sound like my old great-uncle Herschel—whom we loved very much, but who was nevertheless an unimaginative, whining, superior, dried-up old stuffed shirt, who was smelly and had been around too long. We used to call my great-uncle Herschel "the old fart."

I speak metaphorically, of course, of the attitude that you represent and the philosophy GMHC has come to represent. I cannot for the life of me understand how the organization I helped to form has become such a bastion of conservatism and such a bureaucratic mess. The bigger you get, the more cowardly you become; the more money you receive, the more self-satisfied you are. No longer do you fight for the living; you have become a funeral home. You and your huge assortment of caretakers perform miraculous tasks helping the dying to die. I do not cast aspersions on these activities, but I ask you to realize how exceedingly negative this concentration of your energies is. Your words to *The New York Times* only confirm this negativism yet again.

I think it must now come as a big surprise to you and your Board of Directors that Gay Men's Health Crisis was not founded to help those who are ill. It was founded to protect the living, to help the living go on living, to help those who are still healthy to stay healthy, to help gay men stay alive. Mercifully, there are still far more of us who are yet alive. Patient Services were added almost as an afterthought. I do not deny the importance of some of these services, though in most cases I think it inappropriate for you to be providing them. (More on this below.) GMHC was founded to utilize any strength it might be fortunate enough to acquire along the way: to bargain with, to fight with, to negotiate with—to use this strength to confront our enemies, to *make* them help us. This is what political strength is all about. It is *all*.

In this city, our enemies include our mayor and our Department of Health. In this country, our enemies include our President, our Department of Health and Human Services, the Hitlerian Centers for Disease Control, the U.S. Food and Drug Administration, the Public Health Service, and the self-satisfied, iron-fisted, controlling, scientific frankensteinian monsters who are in charge of research at the National Institutes of Health and who, with their stranglehold grip of death, prevent any research or thinking that does not coincide with the games their narrow minds are playing. If, after six years of this epidemic and the years you have been in charge at GMHC, you can view any of these entities or personages as anything other than our enemies, then you are perversely unsuited for your job and should be replaced immediately.

These are a lot of enemies. It would appear to represent the entire "Outside World." I did not believe in 1981 that by 1987 I would sound paranoid; I consider myself to be blessed with hard-nosed, cold sanity, which becomes more objective and realistic day by day.

Most of GMHC's efforts are devoted to providing services the *city* should be providing and would probably be forced to provide if GMHC were not in existence. This is not to say you are not providing them better than the city would; you are. But in taking our money, you are, in essence, asking us to pay twice for what you are doing—once in our contributions to you, and once in our taxes to this city. Thus you should be providing for us additional services our city will never provide—gay services, gay leadership. You don't. You have become simply another city social service agency, and at the rate one hears about your inner squabblings, the rapidly declining quality of the staff you are hiring, and the increasing unhappiness of those who work for you, it will not be long before you are indistinguishable from any of the city departments—Health, Police, Parking Violations—that serve our city so tepidly.

1. AIDS patients in New York still receive care far inferior to that in San Francisco, Los Angeles, Houston, Boston, and Paris (to name only a few cities that come to mind). I would not like to get sick with AIDS in New York and be forced to deal with the lack of decent treatment facilities, particularly if I had no adequate health insurance. How have you let this happen? First-rate health care should be your highest priority. Houston has an entire new and gleaming hospital dedicated solely to AIDS patients. San Francisco, from the very beginning, had entire divisions of hospitals put aside for us. How dare you, your executive staff, and your Board not be the leaders in fighting for these decent treatment centers?

The mayor has seen to it that GMHC has been given just enough money to shut you up. But in buying your silence, this city has lost: coordinated AIDS care, decent hospital care, home care, housing, systematic public education programs, extensive risk-reduction education programs. Through no fault of your own, you are actually perpetuating misery.

2. Your role in demanding better city education has been lackluster at best. You may congratulate yourselves on the many brochures and pamphlets you have distributed, but as you well know, this is like throwing crumbs to only the few hungry birds. Why have you not pressured government, city, state, and federal, to educate more widely? It is appalling that, consistently, year after year, this is overlooked. And it is fully in your province to expedite it. The governments of England, France, Germany, and Norway are mailing to EVERY SINGLE PERSON IN THOSE COUNTRIES full educational infor-

mation, pamphlets with specific do's and don'ts. It is simply puerile and futile to believe that you can educate an entire city and an entire world yourselves with pamphlets and brochures. You can't. It is a gigantic and enormous task. That you do not fight for the education of everyone is a shocking waste of both your energies and an ignoble denial of your charter. How dare you?

3. And just who is it you are attempting to educate? You seem to go at it in such scattershot fashion. You are given a great deal of money to educate everyone, but you overlook with amazing aplomb the vast majority of women, blacks, outer-borough and inner-city residents, children—almost everyone except gay men. It is hard to defend you against charges of racism and sexism. If you are going to cater mainly to gay, white, middle-class males, then you should say so and accept only a percentage of your city and state grants. (Your recent sad and sorry attempt to provide an educational forum for women was a total embarrassment from beginning to end. Much of the best AIDS work in this city and country has been developed by women. Why were so many of them actually forbidden input?)

4. Why have you not been in the forefront of demanding the immediate availability of drugs on a "compassionate usage" basis to those who are in the throes of dying anyway? Even putting aside the (I think untenable) notion that false hope is being provided, the availability of these drugs could provide invaluable efficacy tests. I know few PWAs who are not begging somehow to be on some kind of drug protocol somewhere, anywhere, but who are turned away at every door. How dare you not use your strength and muscle to further these ends?

Why, in fact, are you not fighting for those who would administer drug trials? There are now many treatment modalities that are promising. You continue to pooh-pooh them all—a negativism beyond comprehension to those of us who have seen so many die. You possess the biggest captive pool of people with AIDS in the world. Such studies would be far more valuable than most of the studies you *do*. Why was it left to Dr. Mathilde Krim to crusade

courageously for the release of AZT? How dare you not
have supported her in this cause? And where are you now,
when the government and Burroughs Wellcome have gone
back on their word to release the drug widely, embarrassing Dr. Krim, who had been promised more than she was
given? Why is it that whenever there is a fight for something substantive and controversial (in an epidemic where
everything is controversial), GMHC is rarely to be heard?

Why aren't you pioneering the availability and use of
antivirals as prophylactic treatment for those now carrying the virus? There is enough medical evidence that this
will prove helpful, and each day that a virus carrier goes
unattended is a day his T-cells can be declining. Studies in
this area are desperately important—truly life-saving evidence may lie in their results, but they are overlooked and
ignored by the NIH, by the CDC, by the FDA, and hence
by hospitals and pharmaceutical companies who don't wish
to finance them themselves. How can you be so retrograde
and inhumane in this most important field?

And why isn't GMHC providing drugs that are unavail-
able, actually selling them to the needy at cost? Why must
sufferers fly to San Diego, rent a car, drive to Mexico, and
sneak drugs back over the border like common criminals,
at a cost in money and energy they can ill afford? Ribavirin
once cost three dollars for a box of twelve in Mexico; now
it costs thirty dollars a box. It will undoubtedly increase
now that Mexico knows its true value. Compassionate doctors in Texas and elsewhere are now buying the drug
directly from the manufacturer at cost, picking it up in
Mexico, and selling it to their patients at cost. Why aren't
you providing services like these? So what if this is circum-
venting the law? A lawsuit brought by the government
against you would be the best thing that could happen to
underline the horror of how the FDA is attending to AIDS.
When *People* magazine ran a story on the one courageous
New York gay doctor, Dr. Barry Gingell, who brought
back ribavirin from Mexico illegally, the FDA was roundly
criticized. Confrontation helps! Why are you such sissies!

It is now reported that AZT is going to cost each patient
$10,000 a year when it becomes available. What are you

doing to confront this abhorrent future in which few patients will be able to afford the very drug that might save them?

How dare you ignore issues like these? These are the things you should be doing.

5. Why do you not ride herd on Research—leaving it to others—like the *Native*—to cry out in alarm when obvious false trials are championed and legitimate avenues are ignored? Why have you not pushed for an Office of AIDS Coordination in Washington? Where is the systematic Master Plan promised by Dr. Edward Brandt years ago, when he was head of the Department of Health and Human Services, and promised as well by Reagan, Cuomo, and Koch? How can you be so infernally silent on this top priority?

6. Why are you spending so much of your time, energy, and money on these interminable "Safe Sex" pageants? I find it ironic to find myself asking this. My initial fights with the GMHC Board, which resulted in my being brutally exiled from your organization, had to do with my insistence, and your refusal, to say anything about sex at all. Now you appear to have gone to the other extreme—as if GMHC were a sort of sex clinic to compete with Masters and Johnson and the hateful Dr. Helen Singer Kaplan.

It simply isn't cost-effective to teach eight hundred men how to play with their pee-pees when millions infected are playing with theirs.

7. What has happened to your presence in Washington? There once was a network of AIDS organizations—of which GMHC was and is the richest and most powerful— that hired a lonely lobbyist—though you could afford many more. He's gone, and I hear nothing about his solitary replacement. Of all the areas that demand your strong attention and support, and our money, at the very top of the list is the necessity of establishing a power base in Washington. I have said time and again until I am blue in the face that it is appalling that some 24 million men and women have no lobbying presence in Washington to speak of. How do we expect to achieve anything at all? The smallest unions, the tiniest of organizations, have staffs of

lobbyists, and that is how small-interest groups, minorities, accomplish things. That is how the National Rifle Association is so powerful and achieves results that are anathema to so many. They organize and fight and lobby. They let Washington know they are there. You have the money for this. How dare you not use it?

Again I state what may come as a surprise to you, your Board, and readers, that GMHC WAS FOUNDED TO FIGHT. How dare you not have some sort of political wing, some sort of spin-off that would see to it that lobbying is done by experienced hands? (Three years ago GMHC Board member Bob Diario was supposed to be preparing such a plan. What happened to it? Why is it taking so long?) Every successful charity works this way, finds legal ways to fight, pressure, lobby. You cannot tell me that the Catholic Church is not one of the most politically savvy organizations around, as is the Salvation Army, the American Cancer Society, Sloan-Kettering, you name it. Hiding behind a tax-exempt status (your constant excuse for being so cowardly every time you have to stand up and be counted on any controversial issue—in an epidemic where just about *everything* is controversial!) is simply no longer tolerable. Cardinal O'Connor's got one of the biggest mouths around. And he uses it. Just like Ed Koch. Where's your big mouth? If you haven't got one—get one! How can you justify having sixty case workers on staff and not one lobbyist?

8. Since I left GMHC, your image, your sense of public relations savvy, your visibility, to put it impolitely, sucks. There is not a better way to increase your power than through press visibility. Article after article appears, and there is no mention of GMHC. Story after story, and no longer is it centered, as it should be, on GMHC. Human-interest stories must be created by talented and imaginative public-relations people and press coordinators and planted in the media. It is not a job for one person; it is a job for a number of people. The papers should have GMHC in every single AIDS story, every single day. That is how you become stronger; that is how you get more money from donations and from grants and foundations; that is

how you gain respect and acquire the power necessary to negotiate. That is how you make the mayor provide adequate treatment for everyone in this city. That is how you get the release of drugs to dying patients. That is how you get educational materials provided to everyone, in the mail, on TV. That is how you get TV stations to broadcast condom ads. How dare you not use adult methods to run an adult organization? How dare you not use the rudimentary tools of modern communications to bolster the power you have inherently been handed by the gay community, your constituents. In the past months there has been another burst of AIDS media attention, with many cover stories, many TV documentaries. In former times, GMHC was front and center. I am saddened to see how rarely you are even mentioned now.

You have more than enough money to hire these people. I don't think it's an accident that your public profile has declined. I think this comes from specific Board instructions. It is an appalling choice.

9. Yes, GMHC was founded to fight, to spread information to gay men, and to fight for them. It was *not* founded, believe it or not, to provide Patient Services of any sort. This came later—and it has come to dominate you. It has provided you with the excuse to be cowards. It has provided you with a cover so that you can say, anytime something controversial requires attention: "We are too busy taking care of patients."

The time has come to rethink this devotion. As cases increase so horrendously day by day, there is no way on this earth that you can continue to provide Patient Services to the whole world. Already the quality of that service you are providing is suffering—how could it be otherwise? Soon you will drown and be totally useless.

If you were the fighting organization, negotiating from the strength that our numbers and our contributions have provided you with, you would use these numbers, this strength, this money, to force the system to provide these services. It is no mystery why San Francisco has services paid for by the city. GMHC was founded to fight for these services. Instead, like some hurt little boy, it has cowered in fear, avoided the fight to get them, and decided that "we'll take care of our own, ourselves." Well, now there are too many to take care of, and you must demand help. You must learn how to demand help.

It is no secret that the gay community in New York is not strong. The gay community in New York is invisible and weak. The gay community in New York is, I believe, in the worst shape it has ever been in politically for as long as I have been in New York, ironically just as the Gay Rights Bill has finally passed.

Since we appear to be a community that is incapable of organizing itself with strength, cohesion, unity, or networking, but only one that is capable of dealing with each other in combat, backbiting, and distrust (I am no exception to this), the services GMHC was founded to provide are more essential than ever. You have had millions of our dollars. You have a mailing list of over sixty thousand—by far the largest mailing list any gay organization has ever had.

You are the strongest organization we have, and our only hope.

Numbers and dollars equal power. How are you able, day by day, week by week, month by month, year by year, to deny this power, to ignore the fact that you have it, and to continually hide from it, as a sissy runs away from a fight? I have in the recent past referred in print to your Board of Directors as "a bunch of nerds." Any issue that is remotely controversial is certain to be turned away from your Board's table. I am ashamed of the whole lot of you. I did not spend two years of my life fighting for your birth to see you turn into a bunch of cowards. I did not spend two years of my life fighting to establish Gay Men's Health Crisis to see it turn into the organization it now is.

Get off your fucking self-satisfied asses and fight! That is what you were put there for! That is what people give you money for!

10. You continue to deny the political realities of this epidemic. THERE IS NOTHING IN THIS WHOLE AIDS MESS THAT IS NOT POLITICAL! How can you continue to deny this fact and assert that your role must remain unpolitical?

You have shut out every dissenting voice. You have effectively cut yourselves off from much of the gay community. If anyone doesn't agree with you, he or she is ignored. The list of your victims is endless—strong voices that, were they a part of your organization, would give you more strength and additional power. Because you would not harbor them, splinter groups were forced to take their issues and start their own homes—a splintering that only weakens, only makes everyone less strong. AIDS Resource Center, the PWA Coalition, AmFar, the once powerful and most useful AIDS Network (so sadly missed, now more necessary than ever as you continue to shilly-shally)—these and innumerable individuals are unwelcome at GMHC. Year after year, I wonder when someone up there will be man enough to offer peace—will try to heal the wounds—if only in the name of efficacy.

11. The world needs to know who dies from AIDS. This is essential if we are to underline the horror of what is happening. When Perry Ellis, Roy Cohn, Terry Dolan dies from AIDS, we must not allow this to be hidden or denied. (In the case of Perry Ellis, not only should we not allow the conglomerate that controls his company to put out lies to the press, but we should encourage a boycott of Perry Ellis products to rebel against the shame of their acts, just as we should not fly Delta Airlines now that it has ruled that a gay man's life is not as valuable as a straight man's.)

Why are you not fighting constantly with the Obituary Department of *The New York Times* to see that AIDS is listed as the cause of death, when it is? (The *Washington Post* reported Terry Dolan's death as from AIDS, as did *Newsweek;* the *Times* and *Time* magazine were the liars. Why did you not set the record straight?) And to insist that lovers be identified as lovers—not as one of the battery of stupid euphemisms they come up with. It has been proved that the *Times* will eventually respond to pressure. You are never there to pressure. Every time you keep your mouth shut, you tacitly claim the shame.

12. GMHC is what its Board of Directors wants it to be. Therefore, if any major changes are to be made, they will have to emanate from that holy table.

But GMHC has also placed itself in thrall to forces other than its Board. Somewhere along the line, the organization was completely taken over by Professional Custodians—social workers, psychologists, psychiatrists, therapists, teachers—all of whom have vested interests in the Sick, in the Dying, in establishing and perpetuating the Funereal. You help people to the grave, to face death. GMHC was founded to fight for life. But the fighters have been shut out, banished, as I have outlined above. Why is it not possible to do both!

Now—what can we do?

1. The fighters must be allowed to return. A branch of GMHC devoted to political fighting, to advocacy (if you must find a nice word to satisfy your tax-exemption excuses), must be established immediately and money poured into it. Your mailing list must be used for fighting. Congresspersons respond to the number of letters they receive, as do mayors. Your volunteers must be utilized for these outreach activities. They, too, must cease hiding behind their nurses' pinafores.

Professor Philip Kayal has done excellent research that has uncovered the fact that your volunteers identify their motives in working for you as more humanitarian than political. They must be made to realize that these two are intertwined, that we will have no future for them to be humanitarians in if they are not political. You have more volunteers than any gay organization has ever had. You have so many you cannot process them efficiently. Many are turned away because they do not have social service or welfare skills. You would have hundreds upon hundreds more if there was an arm of GMHC that allowed for advocates and their tactics. How dare you delay this any longer?

2. You must commence a complete rethinking of your goals and cease in your futile attempts to be *THE* AIDS SERVICE AND EDUCATION FOUNDATION. You are uncomfortable providing services to anyone other than gay men; perhaps you should concentrate your services just upon gay men. You have become weaker mainly as

you have tried to take care of everyone. The addict population is the fastest-growing AIDS category, and you are
simply out to lunch in this area. There is nothing wrong in
becoming a special-interest group. Indeed, that is what
you were first established to be.

3. Weed out the wimps on your Board of Directors and
among your staff. Replace them with fighters, with men
and women who are unafraid, who have connections in
high places they are not afraid to use. I am constantly
appalled that at least two members of your Board are on
close personal terms with the mayor, and that this has
produced absolutely zilch in tangible results for GMHC.

4. Begin the healing process. Draw back to yourselves
the splinter AIDS organizations dealing with gay men.
Draw back to yourselves the many in our community that
you have alienated and exiled. Educate your staff on the
history of GMHC, who founded it and what they fought
for and went through to make it the organization you
inherited.

5. I call upon your hundreds of volunteers to mobilize
and discuss what I am writing about. I hear so many stories of volunteer discontent. Now is your chance to make
your voices heard. You are, in essence, GMHC's slaves—
the oil for the Board's machinery—you do what they allow
you to do. But, as with all forms of slavery, the masters
could not exist without you.

6. As for everyone reading this:
We are all exceptionally tired. We are all AIDSed out.
In our exhaustion we allow the tendency to Let Someone
Else Do It. In our exhaustion we foster our continued
ignorance: We don't keep up with what is going on; we
don't want to know. We should read the *Native;* we should
read every article on AIDS. In this ignorance and exhaustion is our destruction. There is no one to do anything but
ourselves, each individual one of us. If the Board of GMHC
has been cowardly, we have allowed it to become so. If
GMHC is on the wrong course, we have allowed it to drift.
If Reagan has not uttered the word AIDS, we have abetted
this. We have given much money to GMHC with the hope
that they would leave us alone, with the notion They

Would Take Care of Everything for Us. But it does not work that way. Yes, they need our money, and will need it now more than ever. But they also need to be told you agree with what I am writing about.

To sum up:

GMHC cannot hope to provide Patient Services for the dying at the rate they are dying, or preventive education for the potentially infected at the rate they are becoming infected. The only way to force the system to provide these services across the board is by political pressure.

Our only salvation lies in aggressive scientific research. This will come only from political pressure. Every dime for research that we've had has come only from hard political fighting.

Thus all our solutions can only be achieved through political action. All the kindness in the world will not stem this epidemic. Only political action can change the course of events.

I challenge you and your Board to lead us. I challenge you and your Board to initiate the process that will bring about your metamorphosis into the organization that will fight for us in all the areas I have outlined above. It is a major challenge and I fear for our continued survival if you fail and we let you fail. GMHC is the only organization strong enough and rich enough and potentially powerful enough. There is no one else. You can no longer shirk your responsibilities, and we cannot let you. I pray that all those reading this will register their support either by writing to the *Native* or to Richard Dunne. I pray that many will agree, that you will not remain silent. I pray that GMHC will respond to this challenge. I am prepared to sit down so that jointly a list of community leaders can be formulated and an agenda drawn so that we can once again attempt to form a united stand against this horrific threat.

I beg the Board of GMHC to hear me. I beg the community of gay men and women in New York to hear me and join me in pressuring for action.

The worst years of the AIDS pandemic lie ahead of us. We are woefully unprepared. There are millions of us yet to die. Please etch this thought on your consciousness: THERE ARE MILLIONS OF US YET TO DIE. Three out of four AIDS cases are still occurring in gay men. Many millions of people carry the virus. Three out of four AIDS cases are gay men. THERE ARE MILLIONS OF US YET TO DIE.

W ith *The Normal Heart* safely launched, and while I was beginning to write several new plays, I found time to start agitating publicly again. And also the energy. In retrospect, I've realized my ups and downs of energy. Earlier I'd always denied any susceptibility to "burnout," but now I see that of course "burnout" came and went and came back again. When it came, I vowed, depressed, never to become politically active again. There had to be others out there to scream and yell; let them do it now.

But it seems that after a rest, my anger always reappears. There was (and still is) no single area of this awful epidemic that is being properly attended to. My list of dead acquaintances and friends grows and grows and grows. More men I once loved, or had sex with, have become ill and died. A continuing barrage of "definite" statements of facts from official authorities are contradicted days, weeks, or months later. I believed (and still believe) little of what I hear to be completely reliable. Anal intercourse was trumpeted (and still is) as *the* most likely cause of transmission. I know too many dead men who could not tolerate anal intercourse. A close friend of mine who has just been diagnosed last had anal intercourse *ten* years ago. That's equally terrifying to me when I read those obituaries of men I'd been with years before 1981.

The above bitter criticism of GMHC came about inadvertently. I received a confidential phone call from a GMHC Board member who was very upset. (The Board had of course grown and experienced a number of changes.) He gave me a list of his complaints, many of which I deal with above. He claimed there was great dissatisfaction among staff and volunteers, and he gave me specific grievances, which I then investigated and found to be true. At first I considered airing these more specifically—mentioning names and slipups. But that seemed to be unwise and petty; there is always backbiting and unhappiness and griping in any organization, and in any event, I realized that the complaints were symptomatic of much larger problems.

GMHC by now was a large and rich organization. I figured they could now withstand criticism and scrutiny I'd been reluctant to air publicly before, when it might do more harm than good. Although Paul Popham and I had not yet spoken or made our peace, I had been told that he, too, was unhappy about most of the matters I raised, particularly the leadership of Richard Dunne.

Paul was no longer actively involved with GMHC. He had been diagnosed with AIDS as early as December 1984, though it was not generally known until the following year, and by then he was quite weak. When this article appeared, I asked mutual friends what he thought of it. I was told he supported my stands almost entirely.

Since his diagnosis, he'd changed radically in his feelings about political actions; indeed, as he came closer to death, he became more impassioned publicly, even going to Washington to testify before congressional hearings. I was proud of him, though infinitely sad that his metamorphosis had come at such a price.

The letters column of the *Native* was filled with responses for weeks. There were the predictable attacks and the gratifying agreements.

There were also to be a few salutary results.

An Open Letter to Tim Sweeney

4 February 87

Mr. Tim Sweeney
Deputy Director for Policy
Gay Men's Health Crisis, Inc.

Dear Tim,

   I am grateful for our recent meeting in response to my *Native* article. It has not been easy for me to reach anyone's ears at GMHC; indeed, when I am asked why I write at such a high pitch of invective, my response is that this seems to be the only way I can get anyone there to hear me. Calmer letters always go unanswered. It is too bad that so often in our community we are almost forced into insult before we hear each other. (Well, perhaps it is like that in other communities, too.) Thank you for being the first GMHC official willing to speak to me in some time. I am sad that your executive director, Richard Dunne, has refused my offer of a meeting and I am sad that your Board president, Nathan Kolodner, has

---

* *New York Native*, Issue 200, February 16, 1987.

not returned my phone call or responded to a similar offer for a meeting.

In any event, I think you and I did good work in preparing a list of six proposals for action. I was thrilled that you agreed with all of them. I was heartened to hear that some of these points are already under development or discussion at GMHC. I was pleased that your opinion of GMHC's Board was more positive than mine; and your assessment that they are indeed ready to forcefully move ahead toward strong, definite acts of politicizing GMHC sounded, to put it mildly, almost too good to be true.

In subsequent conversation with you, I began to feel that my initial enthusiastic reaction to our meeting should perhaps be touched with a little caution. You are only one man, with only the strength of one man—great though I know your strengths to be, and your passion, and your commitment. (I was particularly touched during our three-hour meeting when you spoke so movingly about how much your new job at GMHC meant to you, and the challenges and the opportunities it presented to you.) I know you to possess that rarest of skills—the ability to negotiate and maneuver in difficult and often treacherous waters. I guess I feel that if anyone can help turn GMHC around, it is you. But you cannot do this without the cooperation of your Executive Director and your Board.

I am always amazed at the strong reactions my *Native* articles arouse. I am told by the *Native* that these issues are among their highest-selling. I know that my phone does not stop ringing, that my mail brings many letters, that people stop me in the street. I am overwhelmed with positive support for my stands. It seems to me that I am saying things that must touch a sympathetic nerve in many people. Even if they respond negatively, they do so with the vigor that can only come from some important button having been pushed. I feel that I am saying what many feel but don't know how to say themselves.

As I told you in our discussions, I have been uncertain how best to respond to your letter. I want very much to provide all support to you in your efforts to bring about the vital necessary changes in GMHC's posture. I want very much for my letter, our meeting, the many supportive calls and letters, to somehow serve as some sort of pressure to move your Board and your

Executive Director forward quickly and forcefully and positively.

I have tried over the past weeks to get a consensus from the
many people I have spoken with. I have called or been called by
several dozen members of our community whom I know to be
active and involved. I have called or been called by current and
past GMHC staff, volunteers, and Board members. Quite
frankly, I was amazed at how many volunteers and staff members wanted to talk; what troubled me was how frightened they
were of speaking for attribution, as if some reign of terror
existed in the homeland. Too much of what I found out was
distressing. Some of it broke my heart. The inescapable fact
confronting me everywhere I turned was this: GMHC is definitely experiencing abnormally glaring and traumatic growing
pains.

Many urged me to continue vigorously to pursue my objectives by releasing full details of all this disenchantment. Much
to my surprise, I found myself making the decision that—for
the moment—it would not be productive to get into a screaming
match, or to wash dirty linen quite so publicly as the recent
GLAAD debacle that has wounded that organization, founded
on principles as lofty as GMHC's. As you yourself said, we have
so much hard work and energy invested in our organizations—
we *must* make them work. And I love GMHC as much as, if not
more than, most. After all, it was founded in my living room,
I gave it its name (for better or worse), I arranged for my
brother's law firm to be its legal counsel pro bono, which they
still are, and I gave it two years of my life, full time. I am very
proud that the organization is there partly because of me, and
I am conscious of the many fine deeds it has accomplished over
the years. If I have pain and anger and frustration as well, it
is very much like that of a parent toward a wayward and unfocused child who is not growing up the way I want it to.

Therefore, for the moment, I think it best mainly to put on
record what our six points of discussion were. In this way, the
community has a guide to what you and I feel needs to be done
immediately, and has a yardstick, as well, against which to
measure your progress and that of your Executive Director,
Mr. Dunne, and your Board's progress in bringing these points
into living actuality.

1. Of top priority is our joint acceptance of the fact that GMHC must immediately establish a distinct division that is totally and wholeheartedly devoted to advocacy.

I am aware that there is some indecision as to whether this division should be within the structure of GMHC, as it is presently constituted as a 501-C (3) tax-exempt organization, or whether a separate division must be established with a 501-C (4) structure, which would allow for total political activity under your supervision, but not allowing for tax-deductible contributions. This is an issue that has been plaguing various Boards since GMHC was founded, and I beg that it not be allowed to drag on unresolved any longer. With the new tax laws, as I understand them, tax deductions for charitable contributions are not going to be as meaningful as formerly in helping to reduce the contributors' income taxes; therefore it would seem to me that a 501-C (4) non-tax-exempt division of GMHC should be established forthwith. This would have the further advantage not only of allowing Operation Outreach to function politically, but of allowing GMHC to utilize $175,000 of every $1 million of its (tax-deductible) contributions for advocacy.

I wish there were not so much constant worry about your holy tax-exempt status. You are an organization that should be pledged to obsolescence, not empire.

a. This advocacy division would be staffed with as close to 1-to-1 parity with the client services division, both in staff and volunteers, as possible. In other words, it would be a distinct partner with client services.

b. This advocacy division would have its very own lobbyists, as distinct from the lobbyists GMHC can hire on its own, and the lobbyist GMHC helps to finance via its participation in the AIDS Action Council. You would immediately hire one lobbyist for Washington, one for Albany, and one for New York City.

c. This advocacy division would hire immediately one full-time person whose sole job would be to increase the number of lobbyists in Washington. This person would go around the country working with other gay organizations and gay communities, the goal being the funding by said

organizations and communities of all or part of the cost of
one lobbyist. It costs anywhere from $60,000 to $100,000
a year to fund a good lobbyist in Washington. It would be
no big deal for the gay community in Houston or Dallas or
Philadelphia or San Francisco to have annual fund-raisers
just for this cause. Each city could, in effect, be responsible
for raising the salary of one lobbyist (several years ago,
EEGO—the East End Gay Organization—was considering
doing just this, but somehow it got sidetracked into participating with the AIDS Action Council). Within a year or so,
we could have a group of ten or fifteen lobbyists in Washington and, for the first time in our lives, begin to have
power in the place where it makes the most difference.

d. This advocacy division would have volunteers devoted to increasing the size of the GMHC mailing list. The
more names on a mailing list, the more power the organization has to barter with. I am told the GMHC list is about
forty thousand names, not sixty thousand, as I wrote.
Well, it should be at least a million. There are many ways
to increase a list—from buying other lists to getting letter-
writing campaigns going, getting everyone you know to
add names for this cause.

e. This advocacy division would involve itself in the
many aspects of advocacy—protests, civil disobedience,
organized mailings to members of Congress and government, the forthcoming March on Washington, visible dis-
plays of both coalition and disapproval. The blacks
mounted a very swift and effective march on Koch's Village apartment after Howard Beach. It has been a long
time since our Candlelight March of, was it 1984?

2. Public Relations: Further staff members experienced
in this very special skill should be hired to work with Lori
Behrman (who was a most effective spokesperson on
"Channel 4 News" of February 3rd). Good PR is basically
about taking important people to lunch, making contacts
everywhere, and learning how to use them. It also requires
imagination—dreaming up new angles for stories and not
giving up until they are placed. Money must be found for
such schmoosing-up. Also, GMHC should issue public

statements on every issue concerning AIDS; in every possible article or media mention, there should be a GMHC quote or mention.

That most noble and courageous of protesters, Andrei Sakharov, has proved to us time and time again that, as *The New Yorker* wrote of him, "the main weapon in the struggle for human rights is publicity."

3. Drugs: We talked about the possibility of GMHC plugging into the pioneering and magnificently enterprising San Francisco organization, Project Inform, or providing essentially the same services here. Project Inform has an 800 number (800-822-7422; in California 800-334-7422) where anyone can get the most recently available information on all current drugs and treatments, how and where they can be obtained, and how they are doing in trials, to the best of their knowledge. I am in no way suggesting that GMHC recommend any particular drug or treatment. Results on all present drugs and treatments are still perplexingly unclear. Many patients do better not taking any treatment at all. But it should be a matter of individual choice whether or not someone wishes to undergo a particular treatment. In order for this decision to be intelligently made, the individual should have available to him, with a minimum of fuss and bother, the latest information concerning the efficacy, availability, and cost of whatever is going on around the world. Few patients have the energy, physical or psychic, to be Sherlock Holmes because doctors aren't telling them what they need to know. Your already existing Hotline would seem a perfect place to plug this service in.

4. The addition to the Board of Directors of four or five new members who are politically adept and active and vocal. I am glad to hear from you that you think the Board is now at last ready for political activism; but the truth is that, as a group, the Board is conservative, and unfortunately a conservative board tends to keep perpetuating conservative boards. They keep voting in people just like themselves.

I would like to interject here advice I had from a dear

friend and very wise woman. I called her for advice on all
of this. Her name is Dr. Gloria Donadello; she is a thera-
pist, a Ph.D., a lesbian, Professor of Social Service at Ford-
ham, a director on one of the earliest Lambda Legal
Defense boards, and a member of the advisory board of
SAGE:

"A board is supposed to be the liaison between the
organization and the community it serves. A board is supposed to be the representative of the community it serves.
It is lousy communication, listening only to your own
voice, if differing opinions are not heard. No organization
can be served well that way.

"People who work for an organization or are served by
an organization have to feel they have access to the power
that is running that organization. They are not going to
feel very good about themselves, or about their organization, when they don't. The leadership is making them not
feel good. And you can't expect people who have the least
amount of power to make the changes. For instance, poor
people can't pull themselves up by their own bootstraps.
Power is with those who have the power. If the board and
the executive director have the power, and they don't use
it, it's very difficult for the line workers, or the community,
to make the changes.

"What GMHC is going through—well, it is unfortunately predictable because this happens at about this time
in the growth of any service organization. I don't know
that it can be prevented, but when it is happening, you
must be very much on guard, and aware.

"It is always the danger that the grass-roots organization gets co-opted by the very system it was formed to
make accountable. Social work started out to reform—to
effect social change. Sadly, now, it's all maintenance of the
status quo.

"Part of the answer is to foster a conviction that rests
in a value that the system must be held accountable all the
time. But that takes courage. The organization has to be
willing to stick its neck out. Unfortunately we place too
much value in our society on the status quo. Challenging
the system is a no-no. For instance, an organization says,

'We're now a respectable organization providing respectable services'—but really nothing much has changed with respect to the rights of gay persons. So, in essence, the organization hasn't changed anything."

5. The establishment of a Standing Community Advisory Board. Some modest method must be found for outside dialogue to get the ears of the power structure of GMHC. This is just good simple community relations and, had it existed, there would perhaps not now be such ill feeling about your purchase of an expensive new building.

6. Fund-raisers like the 1983 Circus event at Madison Square Garden. This certainly is not such an important item as any of the first four points, and I offer it more for the morale of the community than for any notion of a cost-effectiveness I know to be less than that of other ways of raising money. But there was something so special about that night at the Circus (the idea was Paul Popham's—GMHC's first Board president) that everyone who attended will never forget it. We could see ourselves in all our magnificent strength—what we were capable of bringing off. How about Bruce Springsteen at Shea Stadium?

At our meeting, I asked you what you thought your timetable might be. You mentioned there were various committee approvals necessary before a full Board vote. Being an impatient sort, I bristled at the notion of committees and lengthy delays. Who among us does not know how often the very process of trying to get anything done gets nothing done? I understand the next full Board meeting is at the end of February.

I look forward to hearing from you about how quickly we can count on a schedule, an agenda, a plan. How long will it take before lobbyists can be hired, this advocacy division established? I hope you will do the community a courtesy by writing a short note to the *Native* to keep us abreast of progress.

AIDS MAY DWARF THE PLAGUE is the small headline that appeared on page A-24 (the real-estate page) of *The New York Times* on Friday, January 24th, 1987. N.Y. AIDS PLAGUE—150,000 DOOMED screams out the headline of the February 4th *New York Post*. "A worldwide death toll in the tens of millions a decade from now" is what Secretary of Health and Human Services Dr. Otis R. Bowen is predicting. His numbers are a bit smaller than those of Dr. C. Everett Koop, the Surgeon General, who says "100 million people could be dead by the end of the century." That 100 million could be infected with the virus within five years is the prediction of Dr. Halfdan Mahler, the head of the World Health Organization. The current issue of *Atlantic* says that for every reported case there are sixty unreported.

I close again, as I did before, with the plea that you, your Board, and your executive director accept this challenge to become the true heroes our community so desperately needs. I close, as I did before, with the startling fact that two out of three official AIDS cases are still happening to gay men. Four million people may now carry the killer virus. The number of new cases is doubling every six to eight months. There are millions of us yet to die.

I do not think that any point or issue I raise in this letter is unreasonable or difficult to put into action. Please beg your Board and your Executive Director not to let us down.

I finally called Richard Dunne and we had a relatively uncommunicative lunch together. However, Nathan Kolodner, the president of the Board, called me and we established a working relationship that has now matured into a friendship. It turned out we shared many similar views of GMHC's problems.

It was to take too long a time, but several new members were added to the Board; they are not as politically forceful as this rabble-rouser would like, but they seem to be committed and intelligent. Lobbying in Washington still languishes, but a New York State lobbyist was finally added. The Public Relations department was modestly expanded, and attempts were made to improve the morale of the staff and volunteers.

Perhaps the most important addition has been the hiring, at my suggestion, of my friend Dr. Barry Gingell, to be head of the new Office of Medical Information. Barry, who is a person with AIDS, knows more about AIDS treatments than anyone else in the world, and he has been an invaluable resource that the AIDS community has come to rely on and revere. He immediately began *Treatment Issues: The GMHC Newsletter of Experimental AIDS Therapies,* which is, I think, as honest and fact-filled a publication as is available on this subject. Barry and a new Board member, Judy Peabody, have joined various NIH drug committees, so that our opinions can at least be heard, if not considered, at that ignoble Valhalla. Of all the voices in all the AIDS bureaucracies, I think Barry's alone has been the most willing to openly criticize and castigate the foul NIH AIDS program headed by Dr. Anthony Fauci, and the equally foul FDA AIDS program headed by Dr. Frank Young, constantly bringing this issue up to the press and at various conferences in Washington, where to criticize the NIH or FDA is to blaspheme God. He has been wonderful.

The Beginning of ACTing UP

On March 14th, 1983, almost four years ago to this date, I wrote an article in the *New York Native*. There were at that time 1,112 cases of AIDS nationwide. My article was entitled "1,112 and Counting," and through the courtesy of *Native* publisher Chuck Ortleb, it was reprinted in seventeen additional gay newspapers across the country. Here are a few of the opening sentences from this article:

"If this article doesn't scare the shit out of you, we're in real trouble. If this article doesn't rouse you to anger, fury, rage, and action, gay men may have no future on this earth. Our continued existence depends on just how angry you can get. . . . I repeat: Our continued existence as gay men upon the face of this earth is at stake. Unless we fight for our lives, we shall die. In all the history of homosexuality we have never before been so close to death and extinction."

When I wrote that, four years ago, there were 1,112 cases of AIDS nationwide. There are now officially—and we all know how officials count—32,000 with 10,000 of these in New York.

---

* Speech given at the Gay and Lesbian Community Center in New York, on March 10, 1987, to a group of approximately 250 men and women.

We have not yet even begun to live through the true horror. As it has been explained to me, the people who have become ill so far got ill early; the average incubation period is now thought to be five and one-half years, and the real tidal wave is yet to come: people who got infected starting in 1981. You had sex in 1981. I did, too. And after.

Last week, I had seven friends who were diagnosed. In one week. That's the most in the shortest period that's happened to me.

I would like everyone from this right-hand side aisle, all the way to the left-hand side of the room—would you stand up for a minute, please? [They do so.] At the rate we are going, you could be be dead in less than five years. Two-thirds of this room could be dead in less than five years. Please sit down.

Let me rephrase my *Native* article of 1983. If my speech tonight doesn't scare the shit out of you, we're in real trouble. If what you're hearing doesn't rouse you to anger, fury, rage, and action, gay men will have no future here on earth. How long does it take before you get angry and fight back?

I sometimes think we have a death wish. I think we must want to die. I have never been able to understand why for six long years we have sat back and let ourselves literally be knocked off man by man—without fighting back. I have heard of denial, but this is more than denial; it *is* a death wish.

I don't want to die. I cannot believe that you *want* to die.

But what are we doing, *really*, to save our own lives?

Two-thirds of you—I should say of *us*, because I am in this, too—could be dead within five years. Two-thirds of this room could be dead within five years.

What does it take for us to take responsibility for our own lives? Because we are *not*—we are not taking responsibility for our own lives.

I want to talk about a few specific things.

I've just come back from Houston. My play *The Normal Heart* was done at the Alley Theatre there. I did not want to go to see it, but a very insistent woman who works with AIDS patients there would not take no for an answer. Thus I had the opportunity and the great privilege to visit our country's first AIDS hospital, which is called the Institute for Immunological

Disorders. I've finally discovered the place I want to go to if I get sick.

You know how the topic of conversation in New York always turns to: Where would you go if you got sick? Which hospital? Which doctor? Quite frankly, I don't want to go to *any* hospital in New York. And I don't want to go to most of the doctors. They pooh-pooh everything new that comes along; they don't know anything about any new drug or treatment. They don't want to know. They throw you into the hospital, give you a grotesquely expensive workup, pump you full of some old drug that they've heard about from another doctor, and your insurance company pays for it, if you're lucky enough to have insurance. These doctors won't fight for anything, they won't go up against the FDA, they don't want to hear about any new theories or ideas. Why are they always so negative about everything? These doctors are making a fucking fortune out of us. They ridicule anything new that comes along, without even trying it. The horror stories emanating from almost every hospital in this city, with the possible exception of NYU, are just grotesque—all the way from an attempted murder of an AIDS patient at New York Hospital to a friend of mine who lay in the emergency room at St. Vincent's for seventeen hours, just last week, before anyone looked at him. No, I don't want to go to any hospital or any doctor in New York.

The Institute for Immunological Disorders is run by Dr. Peter Mansell, who is one of the top AIDS doctors in America. It has space for 150 patients. There are only sixteen patients there. This most wonderful AIDS hospital in the world—you probably don't even know about it; some of you are hearing about it for the first time. How can it happen that it only has sixteen patients? Only in America.

I'm going to tell you—it's not explicitly germane to us, but it is interesting—Texas is the only state in this country where if you don't have insurance, where if you're indigent, the state will not reimburse you or a hospital for the cost of your care. Most of those with AIDS in Houston don't have any insurance. They can't afford to go to Dr. Mansell's hospital. Mansell treats 150 patients every week, as outpatients, for free. Dr. Mansell's hospital, which is owned by a for-profit corporation, is losing a great deal of money. This hospital must not be allowed to die.

Dr. Mansell has found out some very interesting things. He has found out that 90 percent of all AIDS problems are better treated at home, and this includes home treatment for PCP. He has found that he can treat patients for two-thirds less than it costs anywhere else—an average of $11,000 vs. $33,000. He has found that the average length of hospital stay of his patients is ten days, versus thirty days anywhere else. The hitch, of course, is that no insurance policy covers outpatient care. The very insurance companies that are threatening to take away our insurance because we cost them too much won't pay for cheaper treatment. That doesn't make much sense, does it?

But the real horror stories that Dr. Mansell told me have to do with drugs and the FDA. Dr. Mansell has five drugs waiting to be tested. I never heard of four of them. He tells me that each has been shown to prove as promising as AZT was when it was approved. Each has passed what are called Phase One Safety Trials, which show them to lack noticeable side effects. The drugs are called Ampligen, Glucan, DTC, AS 101, and MTP-PE (for KS). He cannot get near the FDA. When one of the top AIDS doctors in the United States can't get protocols through the FDA, we're in big trouble. He showed me the protocols that he submits, and he showed me how they're sent back—the FDA asking for one sentence rewritten, three words revised—nothing substantial—each change causing a delay of six to eight months. Ampligen is a drug that has been around for a long time. Concerned citizens of Houston have formed a foundation and bought $250,000 worth of Ampligen, so neither the hospital nor the government had to pay for it—and the drug remains unused and untested because of FDA quibbling.

You know—each step of this horror story that we live through, we come up against an even bigger brick wall. First it was the city, then the state, then the CDC, then the NIH. Now it's the FDA. Ann Fettner wrote last week in the *Village Voice* about the FDA: "It is a bureaucratic mess, they aren't even computerized, things 'are likely to get stuck in the mailroom,' says Duke University economist Henry Grabowski—which means that much of our pharmaceutical talent diddles with refinements of approved drugs while many that are desperately

needed are put on hold." A new drug can easily take ten years
to satisfy FDA approval. Ten years! Two-thirds of us could be
dead in less than five years.

In 1980 the then head of the FDA said, "Ribavirin is probably the most important product discovered during the intensive
search for antiviral agents." It's 1987 and we still can't get it.
Fettner says, "It's astonishing that ribavirin wasn't chosen
before AZT." Leading researchers I have talked to explain this
one way: The FDA doesn't like the difficult, obstreperous head
of ICN Pharmaceuticals, which manufactures ribavirin, while
Burroughs Wellcome, which makes AZT, is smooth, politically
savvy, with strong PR people. The fast introduction of AZT was
described to me in one word by a leading doctor: "Greed." He
thinks little of AZT, refers to it as "yesterday's drug, that
Burroughs Wellcome is trying to make their fortune out of
before it's too late. I have too many patients on it who are
becoming transfusion-dependent." I have a few friends who
seem to be doing well on it. I have some who aren't. It's certainly not our savior.

AL 721 isn't even a drug—it's a food! How dare the FDA
refuse to get it into fast circulation when it has proved promising in Israel at their famous Weizmann Institute? Indeed,
Praxis Pharmaceuticals, which holds the American rights to it,
could put it out as a food; but they apparently are gambling for
big bucks by waiting for FDA approval to put it out as a drug,
which is going to take forever, because Praxis doesn't appear
to have much experience in putting out drugs at all. Rumor has
it, also, that Praxis has forbidden the Weizmann Institute and
Israeli doctors from giving AL 721 to any non-Israelis who go
to Israel to get it.

What's going on here? To quote Dr. Mansell: "The FDA
makes me froth at the mouth." We have reached a brick wall.
There is a fortune being tossed at AIDS, but it's not buying
anything. To quote Dr. Mansell: "A lot of money, a lot of energy—and very little to show for it." He runs one of the NIH-
designated AIDS treatment centers and he has a hospital with
sixteen patients! And we have ten thousand cases in New York
City. He has an empty hospital, and he is one of the smartest
men in this epidemic. How can this country be so wasteful!

Another researcher: "The NIH is too slow and too

determined to maintain central control. It is hugely bureaucratic, much like your own GMHC and other AIDS organizations have become." Not my words. Dr. Mansell again: "Many
of the drugs that the NIH is testing have already proved useless and ineffective somewhere else. Why do they insist on
testing them? Why do they refuse to test any of these new
drugs that are brought to their attention?"

Let's talk about double-blind studies that we're forced to
endure. Did you know that double-blind studies were not created originally for terminal illnesses? I never knew that. Did
you know that? How dare they, then, make us endure double-
blind studies? They are ludicrously inhumane when two-thirds
of this room could be dead in less than five years.

Double-blind studies are also exceptionally foolish, because
PWAs lie to get the drugs. I'd lie. Wouldn't you? If they told
me what to say to get a promising treatment, I'd say it, whether
it was true or not. I have friends who have forged their medical
records, who have gone to medical libraries to learn the correct
terminology to fill in the blanks. So all the results from all these
double-blind studies aren't going to tell anyone a thing. We're
willing to be guinea pigs, all of us. Give us the fucking drugs!
Especially if Dr. Mansell has five drugs that he says may have
fewer side effects than AZT.

Almost one billion dollars will be thrown at AIDS, and it's
not buying anything that will save two-thirds of the people in
this room. I just heard about a college on Long Island that's
been awarded a $600,000 grant from the Centers for Disease
Control—an organization I have come to loathe—to study
AIDS stress on college students. I can tell them right now and
save the government $600,000. I know what it's like to be
stressed. So do you.

I called up the offices of our elected officials and asked them
to send someone here tonight. Cuomo, D'Amato, Moynihan,
Koch. Every single one of them treated me as if I was ungrateful. "We have been on the front line of getting you your
money," each one of them said. "Leave us alone. You got your
money. What else do you want?" That was from Moynihan's
office: "What else do you want? We got you your money." When
I try to tell them that this money isn't working right, isn't

buying us anything, isn't properly supervised—once again, they don't want to know. I find the offices of Moynihan and D'Amato particularly insensitive to gay issues. Our only friend in Congress, and he's getting real tired, is Ted Weiss. And, of course, from Los Angeles, Henry Waxman.

So what are we going to do? Time and time again I have said—no one is going to do it for us but ourselves.

We have always been a particularly divisive community. We fight with each other too much, we're disorganized, we simply cannot get together. We've all insulted each other. I'm as much at fault in this as anyone.

I came back from Houston and I called people I haven't spoken to in many years. I called Paul Popham. Those of you who are familiar with the history of GMHC and with *The Normal Heart* will know of the fights that he and I had and the estrangement of what had once been an exceptionally close friendship. Paul is very ill now. He and I spoke for over an hour. It was as if it were the early days of GMHC again, and we were planning strategy of what had to be done. We talked not about the hurts that each had caused the other. He supported me in everything that I am saying to you tonight, and that I have been writing about in the *Native* in recent issues. He would be here tonight, except that he had chemotherapy today. He asked me to say some things to you. "Tell them we have to make gay people all over the country cooperate. Tell them we have to establish some way to cut through all the red tape. We have to find a way to make GMHC, the AIDS Action Council, and the other AIDS organizations stronger and more political."

We talked a lot about GMHC, the organization that represents so much of our joint lives. As you know, I have been very critical of GMHC recently, and wrote a rather stinging attack on them. Paul and I both feel that GMHC is the only AIDS game in town in this country, and, like it or not, they have to be made to act stronger in the areas of lobbying and advocacy. There are no other organizations with as much clout, with as much money, with as much staff. San Francisco's AIDS organizations still have not even put their pledged contributions into the AIDS Action Council, our joint lobbying effort in Washington, which is an appalling act on the part of San Francisco's gay community. "We have to shame them into their contributions," Paul said.

The people administering GMHC are running what amounts to a big corporation. We cannot fault them for running such a sound ship, such a fiscally sound ship.

But we desperately need leadership in this crisis. We desperately need a central voice and a central organization to which everything else can plug in and be coordinated through. There isn't anyone else. And in this area of centralized leadership, of vision, of seeing the larger picture and acting upon it, GMHC is tragically weak. It seems to have lost the sense of mission and urgency upon which it was founded—which Paul and I fought so hard to give it.

In my recent article attacking them, I asked GMHC for very specific things: lobbying; an advocacy division; more public-relations people to get the word out; a change of their tax-exempt status to allow for increased political activities; fighting for drugs; more strong members put on their Board. I was promised everything. I couldn't believe it; it was too good to be true.

Two months later, precious little has been done. The tax-exempt status has been changed. A lobbyist has been identified for Albany. A *part-time* PR person is about to be hired. When I asked why they were not hiring a full-time PR person, *six* full-time PR persons, the excuse I was given was "We don't have a desk." Two-thirds of us could be dead in five years, and this rich organization is not hiring people to get the word out because they haven't got room for a desk. [Cries from the audience of "Shame, shame!"]

No advocacy plan has emerged from GMHC, despite the fact that we have been promised one for six months. Paul Popham himself told me that the "Mission Statement" that was prepared by GMHC's executives is one that he never would have accepted when he was president of the Board.

This morning's front page of *The New York Times* has an article about two thousand Catholics marching through the halls of Albany today. On the front page of the *Times*. With their six bishops (including one whom we know to be gay). Two thousand Catholics and their bishops marching through the halls of government. That's advocacy! That's what GMHC has to plan and facilitate and encourage. That's what all of us have to do. Southern Methodist University gets on national television protesting something about their football team. Black people marched on Mayor Koch's apartment only days after Howard Beach. Why are we so invisible, constantly and forever! What does it take to get a few thousand people to stage a march!

Did you notice what got the most attention at the recent CDC conference in Atlanta? It was a bunch called the Lavender Hill Mob. They got more attention than anything else at that meeting. They protested. They yelled and screamed and demanded and were blissfully rude to all those arrogant epidemiologists who are ruining our lives.

We can no longer afford to operate in separate and individual cocoons. There cannot be a Lavender Hill Mob protesting without a GLAAD mobilizing the media, without a National Gay and Lesbian Task Force and AIDS Action Council lobbying in Washington, without a Human Rights Campaign Fund raising money, and without a GMHC and its leaders leading us. That's coordination. Without every organization working together, networking, we will get nowhere.

We must immediately rethink the structure of our community, and that is why I have invited you here tonight: to seek your input and advice, in the hope that we can come out of tonight with some definite and active ideas. Do we want to reactivate the old AIDS Network? Do we want to start a new organization devoted solely to political action?

I want to talk to you about power. We are all in awe of power, of those who have it, and we always bemoan the fact that we don't have it. Power is little pieces of paper on the floor. No one picks them up. Ten people walk by and no one picks up the piece of paper on the floor. The eleventh person walks by and is tired of looking at it, and so he bends down and picks it up. The next day he does the same thing. And soon he's in charge of picking up the paper. And he's got a lot of pieces of paper that he's picked up. Now—think of those pieces of paper as standing for responsibility. This man or woman who is picking up the pieces of paper is, by being responsible, acquiring more and more power. He doesn't necessarily want it, but he's tired of seeing the floor littered. All power is the willingness to accept responsibility. But we live in a city and a country where no one is willing to pick up pieces of paper. Where no one wants any responsibility.

It's easy to criticize GMHC. It's easier to criticize, period. It's harder to do things. Every one of us here is capable of doing something. Of doing something strong. We have to go after the FDA—fast. That means coordinated protests, pickets, arrests. Are you ashamed to be arrested? I would like to acknowledge one of the most courageous men in this country, who is with us here tonight. He is so concerned about the proliferation of nuclear weapons that he gets arrested at the expense of his own career. He uses his name and his fame to help make this world a better place. Martin Sheen. Stand up, Martin. The best man at Martin's wedding, his oldest friend, died today, from AIDS.

Look at this article from the *San Francisco Chronicle*, written by openly gay journalist Randy Shilts (just about the only reporter and the only newspaper in this entire country covering AIDS with proper thoroughness and compassion). Look who is our friend: the Surgeon General, C. Everett Koop. A fundamentalist is our friend. Koop said, "We have to embarrass the administration into bringing the resources that are necessary to deal with this epidemic forcefully." He said a meeting has been arranged with the President several times, and several times this meeting has been canceled. His own Surgeon General is telling us that we have to embarrass the President to get some attention to AIDS. Why didn't any other paper across this country pick up this story? You sure didn't see it in *The New York Times*.

It's our fault, boys and girls. It's our fault. Two thousand Catholics can walk through the corridors of Albany. The American Foundation for AIDS Research has on its board Elizabeth Taylor, Warren Beatty, Leonard Bernstein, Woody Allen, Barbra Streisand, Michael Sovern (the president of Columbia University), a veritable *Who's Who;* why can't they get a meeting with the President—their former acting buddy? Why don't we think like that?

Well, until we all bend over and pick up all those little pieces of paper, I don't have to tell you what's going to happen.

Nora Ephron had canceled at the last moment, and the Gay and Lesbian Community Center asked me to fill in for her at their monthly speakers' series. I had no idea what I wanted to talk about. I didn't particularly want to make a speech at all. I thought I'd said everything I had to say or could say—too many times. There didn't seem to be anything new to talk about.

For the previous month or so I'd been receiving persistent, pestering calls from a charming but determined woman in Houston. Her name was Mary Lou Galantino and she was Physical Therapy Coordinator at the Institute for Immunological Disorders. She simply would not take no for an answer. I must come to Houston to see my play, and I must come to see the Institute. Finally, when she managed to get the theatre to pay my plane and hotel expenses, I gave in. As I look back on it, it seems, like my appointment with Dr. Alvin Friedman-Kien at NYU in 1981, one of those fateful journeys. I wonder, if I hadn't gone to Houston and visited Dr. Mansell's Institute, what I would have spoken about. I wonder, if I hadn't gone to Houston, whether ACT UP would have been founded. Luck has been twice on my side: As with GMHC, I've been able to help coalesce already existing energy that is out there and help find a focus for its outlet.

There was much discussion following my speech, and the result was a decision to hold a further meeting, two days later. The gay grapevine functioned remarkably well, for some three hundred or more showed up that Thursday night, and the result was the establishment of ACT UP—the AIDS Coalition to Unleash Power—an ad hoc community protest group that, originally, was pledged to concentrate on fighting for the release of experimental drugs. (I say "originally" because its interests have now broadened to include other items and I feel they've lost a bit of focus on the drug

issue, which for me is just about the main issue of para-
mount importance.)

A mass demonstration was planned for Tuesday
morning, March 24th, on Wall Street, against the FDA.
Joseph Papp contributed an effigy (built in his work-
shops) of Dr. Frank Young, the head of the FDA, who
was "hung" in front of Trinity Church. Some 250 men
and women tied up traffic for several hours and passed
out tens of thousands of fact sheets about the FDA
horror show, as well as copies of my *Times* op-ed piece
(which follows). The demonstration and subsequent arrests made the national nightly newscasts, and when,
several weeks later, Dr. Young made some promises
(which he has yet to keep) about speedier drug testing
and release, Dan Rather gave credit to ACT UP. It was
a wonderful beginning.

Since then, ACT UP has grown to several thousand
members and has inspired many chapters all across the
country. It often seems that not a week goes by in which
a protest is not going on somewhere. In New York, just
about every possible target has been zapped, and many
of these demos have made the papers and the TV news.

While these two organizations, GMHC and ACT UP,
have given me a certain pride in that I helped to start
them, I've discovered from both experiences that I'm
better as an idea man than as someone easy to have
around after that. The kind of energy that helps start
organizations, and fuel them in the tentative early days,
is also the same kind of energy that becomes embarrassing to organizations once they become healthy, large,
and, in the case of GMHC, bureaucratized. I'm simply
too opinionated, and impatient to move faster. GMHC
became timid very quickly, and my speaking out so
boldly and so violently against my list of perceived
wrongs and enemies terrified the early members. With
ACT UP, there has been a different set of problems:
Everyone is very opinionated, and very angry. When I
found, once again, that what I had learned to recognize,
at last, was my style, was once again going to get me
in hot water (what I have come to call the "fuck the

founding father" syndrome), I quietly withdrew from active ACT UP participation, (although I try to join as many demonstrations as I can). I didn't want to repeat the GMHC experience.

I also now accept, albeit reluctantly, that, once started, there is little any one individual can do to control or affect an organization's development. It's like a person: It's more or less going to be what it's going to be. And, like a person, it wants to do it and get there on its own. And when I found that my suggestions were coming to be resented, not because of their content but because *I* was making them, I returned home to get back to my writing.

ACT UP became strong and healthy very quickly. The group is, for me, infinitely moving to witness, because it is composed mostly of such young people. These are men and women, some barely in their twenties, who have a comfort with their homosexuality that I never had at that age, and a desire to be politically active that, at such a young age, for such large numbers, is actually historically new and important in the ongoing struggle for gay rights.

The FDA's Callous Response to AIDS

Many of us who live in daily terror because of the AIDS epidemic cannot understand why the Food and Drug Administration has been so intransigent in the face of this monstrous tidal wave of death. Its response to what is plainly a national emergency has been inadequate, its testing facilities inefficient, and access to its staff and activities virtually impossible to gain. One private doctor, anticipating the FDA's release of the drug AZT, said that it would amount to a "sop to the gay community—so they'll shut up. They can't say they haven't been given *something.*"

Indeed, these are understatements. There is no question on the part of anyone fighting AIDS that the FDA constitutes the single most incomprehensible bottleneck in American bureaucratic history—one that is actually prolonging this roll call of death. This has been only further compounded by President Reagan, who has yet to utter publicly the word "AIDS" or put anyone in charge of the fight against it.

As cofounder of Gay Men's Health Crisis, America's first

* The Op-Ed page of *The New York Times,* March 23, 1987.

and largest community self-help AIDS organization, I have talked with doctors across the country. Most are reluctant to speak for the record—an act that often jeopardizes their grants from governmental agencies such as the National Institutes of Health, or even further impairs their relationship with the FDA.

But here are some of the things that privately infuriate them:

1. Dr. Frank E. Young, the FDA's commissioner, said that because of new rules and procedures, the FDA might now be able to shave two to three years from the seven to nine years of testing now required before drugs are released for general use. AIDS patients do not have that long to live. In New York City, the grotesque statistics now predict that upwards of two-thirds of all those infected (about a million people in America, according to the Centers for Disease Control) could be dead in less than five years. And it is not just men who are involved. In New York City, Acquired Immune Deficiency Syndrome is now the number-one killer of women between twenty-five and twenty-nine years old, the number-two killer of women between thirty and thirty-four years old, and the number-three killer of women between fifteen and nineteen. Heterosexual women who are not intravenous drug users have the highest rate of increase of any group.

2. Doctors everywhere are waiting to put into immediate use a battery of drugs that have passed Phase One safety trials—that is, drugs that are perceived to have no or few serious side-effects. All of these are considered much less toxic than AZT, which the FDA has now rushed into circulation and which is proving unsatisfactory in many trials, making numerous patients, in the words of one doctor, "transfusion-dependent."

No one can understand why AZT (the brand name is Retrovir) was released Friday, when ribavirin, a less toxic and many think a more promising drug, has not been made available. Food and drug authorities in Britain are preparing to release ribavirin widely.

3. In addition to ribavirin, why is the FDA withholding

Ampligen, Glucan, DTC, DDC, AS 101, MTP-PE, and AL 721? AL 721 is not even a drug but a food—a form of lecithin—that has proved promising at the Weizmann Institute in Israel. Ribavirin, at least, is available at black-market prices in Mexico for those who have the strength and money. None of the other drugs are available anywhere. Doctors wishing to test them have showed me the thick protocols they have submitted to the FDA, only to have them returned again and again with petty requests for the rewriting of one sentence, or the reversal of the order of several sentences, or the elimination of two words.

4. AIDS sufferers, who have nothing to lose, are more than willing to be guinea pigs. If all of the drugs listed here are thought to be less toxic than AZT, and AZT is available (albeit at the unconscionable rate of $10,000 per year per patient), we cannot understand for the life of us, or for what life in us many of us still cling to hungrily, why the FDA withholds them—especially when the victims are so eager to be part of the experimental process.

5. The FDA's continued insistence on double-blind studies (in which some patients receive the drug and others placebos—no one knowing which until the study is over) is incomprehensible.

Double-blind studies were not created with terminal illnesses in mind. It is, again, inhumane to withhold drugs from terminally ill patients willing to take them, Phase One trials having been completed safely. In the past, the FDA has authorized the "compassionate usage" of certain drugs. Why deny the same courtesies today to those with AIDS?

6. Indeed, there is no way the FDA, or anyone else, can set up genuinely "controlled" studies. Such studies require people to certify that they have or have not suffered from certain diseases in the past. But people with AIDS will say and do anything to obtain a drug or join a test. They forge their medical records, and because the FDA bureaucracy is so entrenched, every doctor I know also lies for them.

7. Why is antiviral therapy denied infected people whose immune systems have yet to be destroyed? Why do we withhold treatment and research until people are terminally ill? How many must die before this obvious mistake is corrected?

8. Finally, all of our federal AIDS-monitoring agencies, including the FDA, the National Institutes of Health, and the Centers for Disease Control, perversely refuse to cooperate with each other and with other countries as well, particularly France, whose scientists are making important strides with a fraction of our financial resources.

In its own inimitable and profligate fashion, the United States is hurling hundreds of millions of dollars at AIDS—but in a completely unorganized and unfocused way. A college on Long Island received a half-million-dollar grant to study "AIDS and Student Stress" but NIH-designated AIDS treatment centers are denied promising drugs and in some cases don't even have any patients. This is true at the Institute for Immunological Disorders, the magnificent new hospital in Houston devoted solely to AIDS, which can hold 150 patients but currently houses only eight.

The Institute's director, Dr. Peter W. A. Mansell, is more despondent than ever. His friends have personally raised $250,000 to purchase a supply of Ampligen for him. Dr. Mansell is one of our leading AIDS experts, and has been since the beginning. If he thinks Ampligen is safer than AZT, why can't he be allowed to test Ampligen? If he thinks all of the other treatments I have listed are safer than AZT, why can't he be allowed to use them all immediately? It makes no sense at all.

Our Surgeon General, Dr. C. Everett Koop, a Christian fundamentalist who has turned out to be a man of high honor and integrity, has been quoted as saying he is trying to "embarrass the administration into bringing the resources that are necessary to deal with this epidemic forcefully." He said he has tried to see the President several times—without success.

It's little wonder that the FDA flounders so grotesquely. From the first day of what now has become a national epidemic, the uppermost levels of the federal and New York City governments have chosen not to acknowledge AIDS. And when the histories of the Koch and Reagan administrations are truthfully written, this scandal will dwarf the political corruption in New York and the foreign-policy blunders in Washington. We need humanitarianism from our President and mayor—and heroism from the FDA.

Message Queen

A few years ago, I heard myself being referred to, behind my back: "He's that message queen."

I wrote *The Normal Heart* for one main reason: the world must know about the saddest thing I would ever know. I felt I had an obligation: Because fate had placed me on the front line of this epidemic from the very beginning, I was a witness to much history that other writers were not. That alone would not have forced me to write about it if I wasn't interested in it. But I was and I am, and I doubt I shall be interested in anything else for quite some time. A writer—this writer, anyway—can only write well about what he's interested in.

I don't consider myself an artist. I consider myself a very opinionated man who uses words as fighting tools. I perceive certain wrongs that make me very angry, and somehow I hope that if I string my words together with enough skill, people will hear them and respond. I am under no delusion that this will necessarily be the case, but I seem to have no choice but to try.

I am no longer particularly interested in plays and movies

---

* Speech given at "Epidemic, Center Stage: A Forum on the Role of Theater in AIDS," sponsored by Gay Men's Health Crisis, April 27, 1987, Washington Irving High School.

and books that are not *about* something meaningful and important. I no longer enjoy going to a movie for entertainment or escape. My mind wanders—why are they doing all those silly, inconsequential acts up there? I don't look down on purveyors of entertainment, indeed I envy them, particularly the ones who make millions of dollars from musicals about roller skaters or movies about outer space or the secret of my success or novels about I'll take Manhattan. But I don't know how much longer I have to live, and I would like to devote what time I have left to trying to contribute something more personally meaningful to this strange, perplexing world, filled with so much horror and so many selfish people.

However, I don't think it is the playwright's or the novelist's or the filmmaker's responsibility to deal in ideas or rhetoric or political meaningfulness. These people can express themselves any way they see fit. No, I hold no Marxist views about the creative responsibility, even though I might seem to live by them. I only know that at this stage of my own life, with death so palpable and continuously close, I only have time, with whatever professional authority my years of living and experience have given me, to be—a message queen.

As I said, I have no choice. I've tried, in the past few years, to write other things: plays and screenplays about non-AIDS matters. But I can't seem to. They seem unimportant. Nothing else seems as important as AIDS—and what gay men are living through.

With the exception of Hitler's Nazi Germany, I have never perceived so much utter wrongdoing in my life. Because of this, I can't understand—and have less tolerance for—why every so-called "artist" in the world is not dealing with the horrors of contemporary life—if not homosexual AIDS, then the AIDS of South Africa, the AIDS of racism and misogyny, the AIDS that is Ronald Reagan and Ed Koch and Phyllis Schlafly and Paul Cameron and Lyndon LaRouche and Jesse Helms and Governor Deukmejian and Representative Dannemeyer and Jerry Falwell and our Supreme Court. You do not have to have AIDS to have acquired a system deficient and immune. If writers everywhere were to write about these horrors, then perhaps there would be no AIDS and I would be free, we would all be free, to think about something else.

But most contemporary art has little relevance to the lives we lead. Perhaps that is why I'm not interested in calling myself an artist. I just wish that those who do call themselves artists, or those who traffic in art—the novelists and the painters and the critics and the professors and the rock groups and the *New York Review of Books* crowd and the Yale English Department crowd and all those many, many arts councils and arts endowments and state councils for the arts and commissioners of cultural affairs and the playwright's festivals and that annual joke called the Eugene O'Neill Theatre Center and all the bland dramaturges and committees who choose plays all over the country for their blind audiences in their bleak theatres and the crass men and women who run movie studios and TV networks and national magazines and control the media and all those self-styled expert judges who give Pulitzers and Nobels and Guggenheims and Ford Foundations, and Tonys and Oscars and Obies and Emmys and Grammys—what silly names they all have!—that somehow all of these who call themselves artists or understanding of art would call themselves artists less and become message queens more.

Finally, I would like to acknowledge the irony of both the offering and the acceptance of this invitation from Gay Men's Health Crisis, this now sturdy and entrenched organization that I founded some six years ago with five other men. It is an organization that I am both enormously proud of and enormously ashamed of—if it is possible to feel both so strongly, and it is. How this organization—which was formed to be our chief congress of message queens—can continue, day by day, week by week, month after month, to be more and more subsumed into the very bureaucracy it was founded to fight to make accountable is a particular galling tragedy to its cofounder. I think it is truly appalling that GMHC has invited Ed Koch to speak at its Walkathon on May 17th: that this organization and this community can continue day after day and year after year to kiss the ass of the one person who has done so little for this epidemic and even less for this organization— indeed he is the one person in this entire world who is more responsible than anyone for allowing this epidemic to get so out of hand—is as criminal as his own acts (which still continue; he does not change).

I can only pray—no, prayers are useless, as we all know by now, for there is no God anywhere who could allow such as is now transpiring—I can only hope—no, there is precious little of that left either, particularly for gay men, as day by day we in the gay community continue passively to participate in our own genocide—so what is there left? I don't know. I simply don't know. I can only go on writing what I write, if not as an artist, then perhaps as an historian. We simply must not allow whatever future world there might be to forget the acts of the Hitlers among us who try to destroy us. I no longer feel so certain that we will survive, even with this knowledge. If only each one of us could say to himself or herself: If I'm going to go, at least I'm going to go out fighting. Perhaps—perhaps— we just might survive if only each of you could become a message queen too.

The Plague Years

Tonight, the President of all the American people is finally going to make his *first* AIDS speech.

He will address a fund-raising dinner of the American Foundation for AIDS Research. He will speak on the eve of the Third International Conference on AIDS, which is expected to draw six thousand attendees to Washington, twice last year's attendance in Paris.

He will tell us that AIDS is awful and that it's his administration's No. 1 health priority, hollow assertions that have been voiced by somebody or other in his administration since 1983. He may talk about his new advisory commission on AIDS, about "education," and about testing.

But what will really count is how long and how seriously Ronald Reagan addresses the issues of research and treatment—the launching of an all-out federal war to find a cure for this plague. Even if he mentions these subjects, it is perfectly clear to me that no matter what Reagan says tonight, it's not going to alter the sorry journal of these plague years.

As a Reagan AIDS bureaucrat told me recently: "God help

---

* *Newsday* and *New York Newsday*, May 31, 1987.

149

us with the AIDS epidemic, because the U.S. government won't. Washington, D.C., is not interested in AIDS." The aide spoke in a very low voice—obviously ill at ease. "Why are you so nervous talking about AIDS?" I asked him.

"Are you kidding?" he replied. "If you don't say what they want you to say, you get reassigned to the Indian reservations."

Choose your favorite horror movie:

The World Health Organization estimates that a total of 100 million will test positive for Human Immunodeficiency Virus (the presumed cause of AIDS) in five to ten years. Estimates vary as to how many of the infected will succumb to AIDS, but there's increasing evidence that almost all infected people will fall ill, and the great majority will die.

The federal Department of Health and Human Services says that in three years our annual health-care bill for AIDS will be $16 billion. In a one-year span, full-blown AIDS cases attributed to heterosexuals who aren't intravenous drug users rose from 1 percent of all AIDS cases to 4 percent.

The numbers of AIDS patients hospitalized increased from 10,000 in 1984 to 23,000 in 1985. Fifteen percent of all acute-care hospital beds could be AIDS-occupied in four years (an 800-percent increase over current levels), according to Rodger McFarlane, the head of AIDS Professional Education at the Memorial Sloan-Kettering Cancer Center in Manhattan.

Says Dr. Mathilde Krim, co-chair of the American Foundation for AIDS Research (AmFar): "Everything about this epidemic has been utterly predictable, utterly, utterly and completely predictable, from the very beginning, from the very first day. But no one would listen. There are many people who knew exactly what was happening, what would happen and has happened, but no one of importance would listen. They still won't listen. This is an epidemic that could have been contained. We definitely could have contained it."

But now the AIDS epidemic is seven years old, has killed 20,798 people in the United States alone, is spreading uncontrollably throughout the population—heterosexual as well as homosexual—and will soon bankrupt the American health-care system.

And now Ronald Reagan is finally making a speech about AIDS.

Will he finally explode the myth that most Americans need not fear AIDS?

"A virus does not discriminate. A virus does not know the difference between black and white or straight and gay or male and female," Rodger McFarlane tells each and every class he addresses. "Why doesn't anyone believe that, even now?"

One answer is offered by a congressional aide who deals with health issues: "Never has such a bunch of second-rate people been put in charge of such a first-rate problem."

One of those in charge is Gary Bauer, forty-one, a former Under Secretary of Education, who is now Assistant to the President for Domestic Policy and head of the Office of Policy Development. He has been in his White House office a scant few months and is credited with helping Reagan put on the new makeup that's going to be worn tonight.

Recently, I asked Bauer if there had been a conscious decision to ignore AIDS. "I've never heard of anyone," he answered, "or even seen anybody wink, or even with body language, suggest that—look, if a lot of people die, hey, you know. . . . Now maybe when I'm not around, they let their true emotions hang out. . . ."

I begged Bauer to ask Reagan to consider his place in history, to institute some noble action before it was too late. Bauer's answer was: "I have not seen enough evidence that this is the Black Plague . . . I think only time will tell. . . ."

Why isn't there a forceful, clear-headed administrator in charge of AIDS—of coordinating research into its cause and developing a vaccine against it, and a cure for it, and of educating the public?

"Our belief is that the President is that already, the AIDS czar," is Bauer's answer.

The boss of the several contending government agencies that deal with AIDS is Dr. Otis R. Bowen, the Health and Human Services secretary. His flock includes HHS, the Food and Drug Administration, the Public Health Service, the National Institutes of Health, and the Centers for Disease Control.

It's the CDC that charts the numbers. The CDC's leaps to

conclusions about who was vulnerable to AIDS delayed an attack on AIDS for years. Since the syndrome (it was not yet named AIDS) was first seen in 1980 and first described in the CDC's *Morbidity and Mortality Weekly Report* on June 5th, 1981, the CDC has been the source of continually changing dicta about who is at risk. (First it was gays and Haitians. Now it's everybody.)

I asked Bauer why Reagan hadn't met with Surgeon General C. Everett Koop, the administration figure who is most outspoken about AIDS.

Bauer replied: "I saw a story where Koop was quoted as saying he had not been able to meet with the President. Let me tell you this: Dr. Koop would not normally meet with the President. . . . The fact that Dr. Koop has not met with the President is really not significant, although it's become some sort of symbol of something, I'm not sure what." Koop is a born-again Christian. His insistence that AIDS be dealt with as a medical, not a moral, problem has made him a pariah not only at the White House, but also to his former brethren in Christ who now boycott dinners in his honor.

Reagan has admitted that he hasn't read the forceful AIDS report that he asked Koop to prepare for him and that was published last October, just ahead of the equally discouraging report of the National Academy of Sciences.

It is Bowen who talks to the President about the state of the nation's health. Bowen declined to be interviewed for this essay.

Jim Gottlieb, staff director to Representative Ted Weiss (D.-N.Y.), said of Bowen: "I can't recall anything substantial he has said on AIDS."

The congressional aide I spoke with said Bowen's pet interest is catastrophic health insurance, which would be available only to those over sixty-five or those disabled for more than two years—qualifications AIDS patients don't live long enough to meet. "A messenger can go to the [presidential] well only so often," the aide said. "Bowen has chosen not to carry AIDS."

The next-highest-ranking federal health official is Dr. Robert Windom, the Assistant Secretary of Health. Windom, in office less than a year, had never before worked in Washington, or in government, or directed a large bureaucracy. A successful Sarasota, Florida, internist in private practice, Windom was chairman of the Reagan-Bush 1984 reelection committee in Florida, Georgia, and Alabama. Federal records show that Windom gave about $55,000 to Republican candidates between 1979 and 1984.

Bowen has handed Windom the AIDS crisis. Earlier this month, I asked Windom why more drugs weren't being tested. "We have a task force for that," was his answer. I asked why appropriated AIDS treatment money wasn't being spent. He answered, "We have a committee for that." I asked him about the most talked-about AIDS treatment, AL 721, "I'm not familiar with the details on that," he replied.

Such responses may be why a leading AIDS lobbyist called Windom "just plain dumb." A congressional aide says, "If his IQ were any lower, you'd have to water him." One of his co-workers did describe him as "a warm, affable, back-slapping fellow." Then his colleague sighed, "But he's out of his league."

Next "in command" of AIDS is Dr. Lowell Harmison, who is Windom's Deputy Assistant Secretary for Health and who also declined to be interviewed. One of Harmison's own colleagues explained Harmison's inaction on AIDS thus: "Lowell's philosophical framework is more 'How do we keep the bastards from getting us?' instead of 'How can we maximize our influence?'"

It took the CDC six long years to admit that it was dealing with an equal-opportunity virus. It has taken the FDA the same amount of time to accomplish something positive.

AIDS drugs are to be given "fast-track" attention when it comes to authorizing their use, FDA chief Frank Young announced this month. (It usually takes six to nine years for a drug to be approved.)

Huge drug companies such as Burroughs Wellcome (the owners of the antiviral drug AZT) seem to have an advantage at the FDA. Small, undercapitalized, or inexperienced companies that might be in the possession of potentially first-rate treatments may not get first-rate treatment from the FDA.

An example is Praxis Pharmaceuticals of Los Angeles. Praxis has the world license to produce AL 721, which was developed by the prestigious Weizmann Institute in Israel. It has taken two years for the FDA to take notice of AL 721, which is derived from egg yolks and could just as easily be distributed without FDA approval as a health food.

There's obviously more potential profit for Praxis in waiting to please the FDA; the price of AZT has gone from $8,000 to $14,000 per patient per year in less than four months since FDA approval. Before approval, Burroughs Wellcome had to give the stuff away.

Patients are now so tired of waiting for AL 721 (it's been two years since a favorable mention in the *New England Journal of Medicine*— and supplies in Israel have been mysteriously cut off) that they've had it analyzed, have passed around the recipe from coast to coast, and now whip it up in their own kitchens. A New York group has ordered $200,000 worth of a Japanese knock-off (one kilo, good for about a month, costs $200) and it's now being consumed. Dr. Craig Metroka of St. Luke's-Roosevelt Hospital Center has advised some of his patients to get it wherever they can: NIH trials of AL 721 are at least a year away.

Patients are also learning to duplicate or obtain other drugs that haven't received FDA approval. They include DTC (a French drug), Foscarnet (from Sweden), and ribavirin, on sale legally in more than twenty countries, including Mexico.

There are plenty of other reasons to go drug-shopping. The few drugs that the NIH and FDA have elected to test have either been busts, like Suramin, or, like AZT, have toxic side effects for many.

(Bauer, by the way, didn't seem well acquainted with AZT— which he mistakenly calls "ACT," although it has received more media attention than all other drugs combined.)

It's no wonder that patients have more faith in their own underground information network than in any establishment sources. There is still no official, central, computerized registry of AIDS information. A doctor in Santa Barbara, California, recently lost a patient to cytomegalovirus, one of the many opportunistic infections that afflict AIDS sufferers, according to Dr. Nathaniel Pier, an AIDS specialist. The California doctor could have learned to treat CMV by calling a doctor in New York.

The NIH is currently everybody's least favorite place. *Newsday, The New York Times,* and *The Wall Street Journal* have questioned why some $47 million appropriated a year ago for the testing of AIDS drugs has actually remained unspent, and why nineteen AIDS Treatment Evaluation Units, established with great hoopla almost two years ago, are either not functioning or are greatly under-utilized.

For example, most of the 150 beds at the Institute of Immunological Disorders in Houston, this country's first hospital devoted solely to AIDS, are empty because none of the $47 million has trickled down to Texas. (Additionally, Texas is the only state in the Union that does not reimburse hospitals for taking care of indigent patients. Administrators of the profit-making Houston institute say it's too costly to hospitalize uninsured AIDS patients.)

"The honeymoon with the NIH is over," is how Representative Weiss put it, as his office prepares to instigate through oversight hearings on NIH delays.

The NIH may be in charge of medical research in this country, but it was none too eager to embrace AIDS. One of the first evidences of the deadly syndrome were unusual cancers in otherwise healthy young men. For this reason, the AIDS question was first tossed to Dr. Vincent T. Devita, director of the National Cancer Institute at NIH. (Neither Devita nor his boss, Dr. James Wyngaarden, who is lord of the twelve institutes of the NIH, had time to speak to me.)

In 1981, Devita was in the possession of almost a billion dollars of research money; nevertheless, he decided that the as-yet-unnamed AIDS, which includes such cancers as Kaposi's sarcoma and various lymphomas, really belonged to the National Institute for Allergy and Infectious Diseases (NIAID), which had one-quarter the budget of the Cancer Institute. NIAID's director, then, Dr. Richard Krause, didn't want AIDS either, but Allergies didn't have as much power as Cancer.

Today, major and painful rivalries between the Cancer Institute and NIAID and inside both institutes are hampering the AIDS fight. Two figures at the NCI, Dr. Robert Gallo and Dr. Samuel Broder, have certainly found new meanings in competitiveness. According to one pharmacologist involved, Broder attempted to disparage Gallo's championing of AL 721 (in that

New England Journal report), mainly because Broder, who's in charge of developing new treatments, hadn't noticed it first. This gave rise to the NIH being condemned by the pharmaceutical community for rarely championing anything "Not Invented Here."

It's also said that Broder and Dr. Anthony Fauci aren't on such hot terms either. Fauci is director of NIAID and chief administrator of the nineteen AIDS Treatment Evaluation Units and of AIDS research and testing for the entire country, and no major decision can be made without him. He is being asked to do more than any human is capable of doing, with predictably human results.

He works eighteen-hour days; he must summon committees, preside over meetings, supervise the selection of drugs to test, monitor their results, deal with pharmaceutical companies, keep up on all the latest information (a new drug application can run to 100,000 pages of evidence), attend conferences all over the world, and put up with complaints from absolutely everyone.

Instead of screaming and yelling for help as loudly as he can, he tries to make do, to negotiate quietly.

Only after intense questioning does Fauci quietly admit that he desperately needs "somebody to cut through all the government red tape." But he doesn't want a larger research staff. "I've got no place to put them," he explained.

It is apparently *verboten* for a new lab to be built on the supremely manicured campus of NIH.

It should also be noted that the beds in Fauci's AIDS ward are, save two, empty. A whole floor in America's state-of-the-art hospital, $47 million given him to fund the testing of new treatments, and his beds are empty! Critics charge that Fauci is so in love with AZT, which he administers on an outpatient basis, that he is not interested in testing other drugs.

The battling over who's going to get the credit in the AIDS fight extends to the international arena. French scientists at the Pasteur Institute announced that they had isolated "the AIDS virus" and developed a test to detect it during 1983. A year later, NCI's Gallo claimed the same discovery as his own.

A recent British television documentary questioned the

honesty of Gallo's assertions and research. The Granada TV documentary also said: "The effects of the row are far-reaching. Senior scientists are refusing to talk to one another. Laboratories fear to exchange samples without watertight legal guarantees. The search for a cure has inevitably been set back."

The bitter U.S.-French dispute over "the AIDS virus" discovery was resolved in March with an agreement to share the patents for the AIDS blood test. But the bitter aftertaste lingers on the international scene, and few European scientists will attend this week's NIH-sponsored meetings.

Dr. Don Francis, a CDC scientist who was reassigned from the CDC headquarters in Atlanta, after criticizing Gallo, told Granada TV that the fight "has truly inhibited the progress necessary to combat this really, really dangerous virus that's now all over the world. Now there are two camps that are divided and therefore make the field a relatively unpleasant one to get into—and that keeps some of the best scientists out."

"You have smart men out there," said Dr. Krim, of the American Foundation for AIDS Research, "who know certain things are not working at the NIH; but it's difficult to expect an investigator to bite the hand that feeds him—the NIH."

Outspoken AIDS doctors have a difficult time at institutions beyond NIH, too. Take the case of Dr. Michael Gottlieb, AmFar's co-chair. Gottlieb, who has been working with AIDS since 1980, recently quit a full-time post at UCLA because, he said, he couldn't obtain tenure. The university claims he resigned before a tenure decision was reached.

The quality of NIH research and American research overall can be judged by the recognition that most AIDS breakthroughs have come from abroad: the discovery of "the virus" at the Pasteur Institute in Paris; the discovery of a second (West African) AIDS virus at the Pasteur Institute; the vaccine studies and experiments under way by Dr. Daniel Zagury at the University of Paris; the possible genetic predisposition toward AIDS susceptibility announced in London by Dr. Anthony Pinching; AL 721 from Israel; CSF, a new immune-stimulating drug, controlled by Sandoz, a Swiss company; and, indeed, AZT itself. Although American-discovered, it is now owned by Burroughs Wellcome, a British bunch.

Who is fighting all this American inertia?

Only two elected officials in Washington sounded the alarm early and have been courageous enough not to run away: Representatives Henry Waxman (D.-Calif.) and Ted Weiss. They've been joined by Senator Lowell Weicker (R.-Conn.)

Senators Daniel Patrick Moynihan and Alfonse M. D'Amato, as elected representatives of New York, the state most under siege by AIDS, have betrayed their constituents by the banality of their response. Nor has the occupant of Gracie Mansion been a Profile in Courage. "It is disgraceful that the mayor of New York does not provide sufficient leadership on this issue," says Nathan Kolodner, president of Gay Men's Health Crisis.

Edward I. Koch was so roundly booed at the recent GMHC Walkathon (which raised $1.6 million to help defray costs of services the city should be providing but isn't) that he ripped up his speech and sat glaring out at the audience, facing signs that proclaimed him THE WORST. WOULD YOU TRUST THIS MAN? one of the signs under his picture asked.

The city recently announced that it has drafted, but not implemented, a five-year plan to deal with AIDS by expanded care for those already afflicted, promotion of research, and expansion of education programs and voluntary testing.

This sounds like the plan Koch announced three years ago that never happened.

Reagan will talk tonight about mandatory testing and "education," and there will be much yelling and screaming from opponents and supporters of both.

It is imperative that the American people realize that while all the heat and fury from the religious right and its equally vocal supporters on the political right continue about the naughtiness of condoms and sex education and homosexuality and intravenous drug use, the presumptive virus continues to spread and kill.

Every stalling tactic costs lives.

They *know* this. Anyone who has watched the numbers of dead grow and grow knows this.

The record convinces me that no matter what Reagan says tonight, no substantial battle for a cure will be mounted while he is in office. There's only one word to describe his monumental disdain for the dead and dying: genocide.

In April 1987, the thought occurred to me that I could perhaps best put my writing skills and my knowledge of the AIDS epidemic to optimum use by writing a regular column, "Journal of the Plague Years." I submitted this proposal to Max Frankel at *The New York Times*, Robert Gottlieb at *The New Yorker*, and David Laventhol (an old childhood and college friend), the president of the enormous Times-Mirror newspaper empire. Frankel turned me down, which was to be expected, but Bob Gottlieb and David both were interested in proceeding. While vanity urged me to accept *The New Yorker*, I thought that being syndicated by the huge *Los Angeles Times–Washington Post* network of newspapers, which is what David was offering, presented the best opportunity of reaching a big audience in the fastest way. Hence I accepted their offer, went to Washington to research the article, came back to New York, wrote it, submitted it, had it edited to shreds of its former self—and then became bitterly disillusioned as it was turned down by every single one of the over three hundred papers the *Los Angeles Times–Washington Post* Syndicate telexed it to, *twice*—including David's own flagship, the *L.A. Times* itself.

The unedited version of the article I submitted, with the tone I was hoping to be allowed in print (magnified now a few decibles higher), forms the core of the speech I made in Boston, which is included as the next piece.

Reagan's first AIDS speech was received with boos. There were many of us in that audience who sat there listening, waiting for him to say something, anything, of import. It was not enough of a gesture for us that he was just *there*, for which we'd been told we must be grateful. He did not use the word "gay" or "homosexual" once. He praised heterosexual AIDS service organizations, but he could not say "Gay Men's Health Crisis." He announced that he was in favor of mandatory testing (the first round of booing), particularly for

marriage-license applicants, prisoners, and immigrants
(the second round of booing), and then he finally sat
down (the final cascade of booing). He'd not said one
word about *doing* anything positive. Elizabeth Taylor,
who had introduced him and who, word has it, was instrumental in getting this stupid man to address this
evening sponsored by the organization of which she is
co-chair, was obviously embarrassed and attempted to
make nice. But Reagan's face told it all. He is not accustomed to being booed in public and he was mad. Dr.
Mathilde Krim, AmFar's other co-chair, who had stated
beforehand that she would walk off the stage if Reagan
recommended mandatory testing, stayed put.

When he spoke at the opening ceremonies the next
day of the Third International AIDS Conference at the
Washington Hilton, George Bush was booed even
louder. "It's those gay activists," he was heard to say.
Well, a lot of it certainly was. But a lot of it certainly
wasn't. At last.

I'd no sooner arrived in Washington to begin researching the above article than I received word from
our mutual friend Craig Rowland that Paul Popham had
just died in Sloan-Kettering. And that *The New York
Times* was hedging on writing a special obituary, complete with photograph. I called Max Frankel's office and
found myself yelling and threatening that if this man
was not properly honored I would do everything in my
power to bring down the wrath of the entire gay community on *The New York Times* forever. Many others also
called, and Paul was given a short, obviously grudging,
few inches, with a photograph.

Then I sat down and, as so often happens these days,
tried to cry. There aren't any tears left. Only infinite
sadness. For all our losses. For the tragedy of all our
fights. For lost friends and lost friendships and lost
opportunities. At least I was grateful that Paul and I
had spoken, as friends, twice more in the past few
weeks, from his deathbed. We both apologized for all
the hurts we'd caused each other. His mind wandered in
and out, and the silences were long between his

thoughts. He repeated himself. "Keep fighting." "Keep fighting." "Keep fighting."

And so the man with whom I had spent so many of the early hours and days and months and years of this horrible plague fighting, too often with each other, to make GMHC a reality, was gone.

I Can't Believe You Want to Die

Weₑ have little to be proud of this Gay Pride Week.

One by one, we are being picked off by the enemy.

They are killing us.

I don't think you are going to like what I am going to say. It is the last time I am going to say it. I'm making a farewell appearance. I am not overly tired. I am certainly not suffering from burnout. I have a lot of piss and vinegar left in me—too much, in fact. No, I'm not tired.

Not physically tired, at any rate. I am, of course, as are you, very tired of many things. I am tired of what *they* are doing to us. I am tired of what *they* aren't doing for us. I am tired of seeing so many of my friends die—I'm exceptionally tired of that, as I know you are too.

I'm also tired of people coming up to me on the street and saying, "Thank you for what you're doing and saying." They mean it as a compliment, I know. But now I scream back, "Why

---

* Speech delivered on June 9, 1987, to the Boston Lesbian and Gay Town Meeting, held in Faneuil Hall, to kick off their Gay Pride Weekend. It was reprinted in many of the major gay newspapers across the country.

162

aren't you doing it and saying it, too?" Why are there so few people out there screaming and yelling? You're dying too!

I'm telling you they are killing us! We are being picked off one by one, and half the men reading this could be dead in five years, and you are all still sitting on your asses like weaklings, and therefore we, the gay community, are not strong enough and our organizations are not strong enough and we are going to die for it!

I have come to the terrible realization that I believe this gay community of ours has a death wish and that we are going to die because we refuse to take responsibility for our own lives.

Yes, most of all, I'm tired of you. I'm tired of the death wish of the gay community. I'm tired of our colluding in our own genocide. I'm tired of you, by your own passivity, actively participating in your own genocide.

How many of you have given a thousand dollars or more at any one time to any gay organization or gay charity? Ten thousand? (For the rich readers: one hundred thousand dollars? A million?)

How many of you have left anything in your wills to anything gay?

How many of you have spent at least one hour a week volunteering for a gay organization? Ten hours?

And if you don't like any of the gay organizations, how many of you have spent how much time to make any of them better? Instead of just bitching them into further weakness? Or helped them raise money to make themselves better?

How many of you have bothered to consider that by helping to raise $80,000 a year, you could fund a lobbyist in Washington to fight for us all year long—to join with a network of other gay lobbyists, paid for by groups in other cities, so that we could have as many lobbyists as General Motors or the National Rifle Association or the National Council of Churches or the American Medical Association, all of whom get what *they* want?

Is it such a big deal to get a group together to raise $80,000 to save your lives? (Did anyone notice that when Paul Popham died, he asked that contributions be made to AIDS Action Council, a lobbying group, and not Gay Men's Health Crisis, which he cofounded, and in whose ability to do anything but look after funerals he had lost confidence and faith?)

How many of you have written consistently or even irregularly to an elected official or testified at an official hearing on the subject of AIDS, or regarding treatment, or official lethargy in this city and state and country?

How many of you really trust the NIH to be capable of coordinating research around a crisis of this scope?

How many of you even know what the NIH is, or how important it is in your life? And that your very own life is in its hands? You didn't know that, did you? That your very own life is in the hands of an agency you don't know anything about.

How many of you believe there is sufficient education to contain what is happening?

How many of you have children? How many of you have spoken to a school board about sex education?

How many of you have had sex with more than one person in the last ten years?

How many of you have protested actively against mandatory testing?

How many of you are willing to face up to the fact that the FDA is fucked up, the NIH is fucked up, the CDC is *very* fucked up—and that, entering the seventh year of what is now a pandemic, the boys and girls running the show at these organizations have been unable to make whatever system they're operating work?

How long are you prepared to wait for these systems to work?

How long are you prepared to wait before our own AIDS organizations provide us with adequate information on available treatments?

How many hours and days are you prepared to spend on the phone attempting, in vain, to find out what is going on where and how it's doing and why your dying friends can't get it immediately?

How many of you believe you have no responsibility to take action on any of these matters?

How many of you need to die or become infected before you feel you can take action on why every single branch of govern-

ment in charge of AIDS, both local and federal, is dragging its
ass?

What's the number of dead friends at which you can decide
to stop just sitting quietly like the good little boys and girls we
were all brought up to be—and start taking rude, noisy, offensive political action? One? Ten? *One hundred?*

It always amazes me when I tell people they have power,
and they answer me, "Power? Me? What power?" How can you
be so conservative, dumb, blind? You know what is going on
better than anybody, and yet you are silent, you constantly,
consistently, and continuously sit on your collective asses and
refuse to use your power.

Your voice is your power! Your collective voices! Your group
power! Your political power! Your names all strung together on
one long list is your power. Your bank accounts are your power,
if you weren't all so devastatingly stingy when it comes to
funding anything gayer than a Halloween costume. Your bodies are your power, your *living* bodies all strung together in
one long line that reaches across this country and could reach
to the moon if we only let it.

You know that this country is not responding on a national
political level or a local political level, and yet you sit by along
with everyone else and watch our men being picked off one by
one by one by one.

No one is in charge of this pandemic, either in this city or
this state or this country! It is as simple as that. And certainly
no one who is compassionate and understanding and knowledgeable and efficient is even anywhere near the top of those
who are in charge. Almost every person connected with running the AIDS show everywhere is second-rate. I have never
come across a bigger assortment of the second-rate in my life.
And you have silently and trustingly put your lives in their
hands. You—who are first-rate—are silent. And we are going
to *die* for that silence.

You know, it's not even a question of government funding
anymore. For six long years we fought so hard to get the
money. Finally Congress has appropriated masses of money.
Can you believe me when I tell you that it is not being spent?
Two years ago, nineteen official AIDS treatment centers, called

ATEUs (AIDS Treatment Evaluation Units), were set up by the NIH—and they still aren't being utilized beyond a fraction of their humane possibilities and intentions. One year ago the NIH was given $47 million just for testing new AIDS drugs—*and they aren't spending it!* Why didn't we know that? Where have we been for these long two years? Why didn't we know that this precious, precious time—during which how many dear friends of ours died—was being thrown out in the garbage because we didn't get on the phone and inquire politely: "Please, sirs, can you tell me what you're doing with all that nice money Congress gave you last May?" How could we have been so lazy and irresponsible—and *trusting?* We, of all people in this world, should know better, and know how not to trust. Where were our gay leaders? Where were all our AIDS organizations? Where were our people in Washington? Where was I? For I blame myself more than I blame anyone else. God fucking damn it, I trusted too!

When I found out about three months ago that $47 million was actually lying around not being used when I knew personally that at least a dozen drugs and treatments just as promising as AZT and in many cases much less toxic were not being tested and were not legally available to us, I got in my car and drove down to Washington. I wanted to find out what was going on. Like most people, I have no notion of how the system works down there, who reports to whom, which agency is supposed to do what. What I found out sent me into as profound a depression as I have been in since this epidemic started.

My first meeting was at the White House, with the President's Domestic Policy Adviser, Gary Bauer, who advises Ronald Reagan on AIDS. I asked him if ignoring AIDS was intentional. He answered me that he had not seen enough evidence that the Black Plague was going on yet. He was particularly interested to hear from me that the current evidence indicates that the gay male population of the major cities is on its way to becoming totally exposed to the virus. He asked me if I thought female-to-male transmission was as potent as male-to-male. I said the statistics were about the same. He said his advisers told him otherwise. I asked him if gay people who were AIDS experts could be on the President's Commission, and he told me No. I asked him why the President had refused to put anyone in charge—to appoint an AIDS czar? He told me the President *was* the AIDS czar. I asked him why the President had not only not read Surgeon General Koop's AIDS report, or the National Academy of Sciences AIDS report—both of which were then over six months old and both of which beg for immediate, all-out action—but he hadn't even met with Koop personally, his own Surgeon General, and he answered me that the chain of command dictates that, in matters of health, the President talks only to his Secretary of Health and Human Services, Dr. Otis R. Bowen. It turns out that Dr. Koop has absolutely no power; his position is simply that of figurehead. They do not like what he is saying, and I think that if you listen to what he is beginning to say now, you will see that Dr. Koop is being pulled back into line.

Dr. Otis R. Bowen would not see me. He is Reagan's *third* Secretary of Health and Human Services, and he is supposed to be in charge of AIDS. Until he appeared as the closing speaker at the Third International AIDS Conference, where I am happy to say he was roundly booed—were any of *you* there to boo him?—he had not been heard to say anything substantial at all about AIDS. The Secretary of the main department of your government in charge of AIDS—the one single man who can report to the President on the state of this nation's health— had yet to be heard saying anything about AIDS, at the beginning of the seventh year of this pandemic.

I discovered that Dr. Bowen had passed the AIDS buck over to his Assistant Secretary of Health and Human Services, Dr. Robert Windom. Dr. Windom has been in his job all of one year. He's never worked in government before. He was a private physician in Sarasota, Florida, and I figure he got his wonderful opportunity to work so close to his idol, Ronald Reagan, by contributing $55,000 to Republican candidates between 1979 and 1984. He is exceptionally ill-informed about AIDS. On a recent NBC Radio coast-to-coast call-in show, he answered two of his questions incorrectly. My favorite description of Dr. Windom comes from a top legislative congressional aide: "If his IQ were any lower, you'd have to water him."

You laugh—and Dr. Windom is in charge of your life! An uncaring, dumb stooge who knows next to nothing about any of the drugs or treatments or research is in charge of your life, and you are laughing! Over half the men here could be dead in less than five years, and you are laughing at this crack about Dr. Windom!

Dr. Windom reports to Dr. Bowen who reports to the President.

Dr. Windom has passed the AIDS buck to his assistant, Dr. Lowell Harmison. Dr. Harmison is sort of the power behind the power behind the throne. Dr. Harmison does not like gays. Dr. Harmison has been described to me by several congressional contacts as "evil." "You cannot say enough bad things about Lowell Harmison," I was told by more than one. He is so frightened of gay people that he was terrified we would intentionally give blood in order to pollute the nation's blood supply—*on purpose.*

Dr. Harmison reports to Dr. Windom who reports to Dr. Bowen who reports to the President.

Bauer, Bowen, Windom, Harmison. These are the four top men in charge of AIDS in the United States government, the government of all the American people. Your government. God (if there is one) help us—because these four idiots won't.

I am here to tell you that I know more about AIDS than any of these four inhumane men, and that any one of you here who has AIDS or who tends to someone with AIDS, or who reads all the newspapers and watches TV, knows more about AIDS than any of these four monsters. And they are the four fuckers who are in charge of AIDS for your government—the bureaucrats who have the ultimate control over your life.

Next I went to the National Institutes of Health. The National Institutes of Health receives $6.2 billion *each and every year* to look after the health of the American people. "To improve the health of the American people" is how the U.S. Government Manual describes the NIH's mission. How many of you can tell me the name of the head of NIH?

You don't know the name of the man who is given $6.2 billion each and every year to help make you better if you have AIDS? You should be ashamed of yourselves.

His name is Dr. James Wyngaarden, and he has never been heard to speak out publicly about AIDS either. He is given $6.2 *billion* every year, and not only doesn't he speak out about AIDS, but you don't even know his name!

Dr. Wyngaarden reports to Dr. Windom who reports to Dr. Bowen who reports to the President.

The NIH is like a college campus. It looks like Amherst, or like something from an old MGM musical. It's really made up of twelve institutes, which are sort of like dorms, or fraternities, all part of the whole. The grounds are manicured and you can't see any shit on the ground.

Seven years ago, when AIDS was first noticed, and you would have thought NIH would jump on it fast, this is what happened. You would have thought that because there was a cancer involved, called Kaposi's sarcoma, it should have gone to the institute in charge of cancer, the National Cancer Institute of the National Institutes of Health. The National Cancer Institute is the richest fraternity at NIH. In 1981, when AIDS first showed up and should have gone into this rich fraternity, the head of this fraternity didn't want it. So he blackballed it. He had $1 billion of research money "to improve the health of the American people," and the head of NCI didn't want it. Now, how many of you can tell me the name of the head of NCI, then and now?

The man who is in charge of the most important cancer research institute in the entire world—and you don't know his name? You should be ashamed of yourselves.

His name is Dr. Vincent T. Devita. In 1981 he didn't want AIDS, he didn't like the smell of it, and he didn't want to spend any of his institute's $1 billion a year on it, so he too passed the buck.

Dr. Devita reports to Dr. Wyngaarden who reports to Dr. Windom who reports to Dr. Bowen who reports to the President.

Dr. Devita passed the buck to a poor relation, a much smaller institute named the National Institute for Allergy and Infectious Diseases of the National Institutes of Health, which had a budget one-fourth of his and which was not nearly so popular a fraternity to rush and was then run by a man named Dr. Richard Krause, who didn't want AIDS either. He must have smelled the shit about to hit the fan because he quickly resigned as head of NIAID, and he was replaced by—now I am sure you can tell me the name of the man who is now the director of NIAID, the man who reports to Dr. Wyngaarden who reports to Dr. Windom who reports to Dr. Bowen who reports to the President—the single most important name in AIDS today, the name of the man who has probably more effect on your future than anybody else in the world.

How many of you know this man's name?

His name is Dr. Anthony Fauci. He's real cute. He's an Italian from Brooklyn, short, slim, compact; he wears aviator glasses and is a natty dresser, a very energetic and dynamic man. After a recent meeting a bunch of us from New York had with him, during which absolutely nothing was accomplished, he asked me what we thought of the meeting. I told him: "Everyone thought you were real cute." And he blushed to his roots.

You are smiling, and this is the man who has more effect on your future than anyone else, and he is not spending that $47 million—*which was given to him specifically to test AIDS drugs*—and you are smiling!

Everybody likes Dr. Fauci and everybody thinks Dr. Fauci is real cute and every scientific person I spoke to whispers off to the side, "Yes, he's real cute, but he's in way over his head."

Dr. Fauci is an ambitious bureaucrat who is the recipient of all the buck-passing and dumping-on from all of the above. He staggers, without complaint, under his heavy load. No loud-mouth Dr. Koop he.

Dr. Fauci, with his devoted staff of several dozen—that's right, folks, no more than a couple dozen doctors and scientists are fighting against AIDS at NIAID; I guess $47 million doesn't buy what it used to—is chief administrator of the nineteen AIDS-designated treatment units around the country, called ATEUs, and of all AIDS research and testing for the entire country, and no major decision can be made without him. He works eighteen-hour days, his wife is an AIDS nurse in his hospital, he must summon committees, preside over meetings, supervise the selection of drugs to test, monitor their results, deal with pharmaceutical companies, keep up on all the latest information, attend conferences all over the world, and put up with complaints from absolutely everyone.

Dr. Fauci, of all the names in this article, is certainly not the enemy. Because he is not, and because I think he does care, I am even more angry at him for what he is not doing—no matter what his excuses, and he has many.

Instead of screaming and yelling for help as loudly as he can, he tries to make do, to make nice, to negotiate quietly, to assuage. An ambitious bureaucrat doesn't make waves. Yes, Dr. Fauci reports to Dr. Wyngaarden who reports to Dr. Windom who reports to Dr. Bowen who reports to the President.

Dr. Fauci has had this $47 million for a year, and worse—the beds in his AIDS wards are empty! A whole floor in America's state-of-the-art hospital, $47 million given him to test new treatments, and his beds are empty, just as the majority of places on the treatment protocols at those nineteen ATEUs around the country are empty.

What the fuck is going on here? Are they actually afraid they might learn something that might save us?

Research at NIH? I have not space to go into the gory details. Let me just say that the research rivalries in and among *all* the institutes at NIH could make a TV series to rival "Dynasty" and "Falcon Crest" in competitiveness, hostility, selfishness, and greed. (Why doesn't the press write about these scandals as they do about all others? Why doesn't the press ever investigate NIH? Is it so holy—like the Vatican?)

Now you know why NIH stands for Not Interested in Homosexuals.

What the fuck is going on here, and what the fuck are you doing about it?

If I use gross language—go ahead, be offended—I don't know how else to reach you, how to reach everybody. I tried starting an organization: I cofounded GMHC, which becomes more timid as it becomes richer day by day. I tried writing a play. I tried writing endless articles in the *Native* and *The New York Times* and *Newsday* and screaming on "Donahue" and at every TV camera put in front of me. I helped start ACT UP, a small bunch of too few very courageous people willing to make rude noises. I don't know what else to do to wake you up!

I will tell you something else to try to wake you up: If AIDS does not spread out widely into the white, non-drug-using, heterosexual population, as it may or may not do, then the white, non-drug-using population is going to hate us even more—for scaring them, for costing them a fucking fortune, for our "lifestyle," which they will say caused this. AIDS will stay a disease of blacks and Hispanics and gays, and it will continue to be ignored, it will be ignored even more.

The straight world is scared now because they're worried it's going to happen to them. What if it doesn't? Think about that for a while. If all this lethargy is going on now, think what will happen then—just as you are coming down with it and facing death.

Who is fighting back in any and all of this? Twenty-four million gay men and lesbians in this country, and who is fighting back? We have a demonstration at the White House and we have three hundred people and we think we're lucky! We get our pictures in all the magazines and newspapers for one or two days and we feel real proud. Sixty thousand Catholics march in Albany. Two hundred fifty thousand Jews march in New York against the treatment of Soviet Jews. One million people march for nuclear disarmament.

What does it take to get you off your fucking asses?

"You want to die, Felix? Die!" That's a line from *The Normal Heart.* In his immense frustration, Ned Weeks yells it at his dying lover. That's how I feel about all of you.

What does it take to make people hate? I hate Ed Koch because he is the one person in this entire world who could have done something in the beginning and didn't and it took us almost two years even to get a meeting with him (we must always remember that, as Dr. Mathilde Krim tell us, "this is an epidemic that could have been contained"), and he has put yet another powerless wimp in place as his Commissioner of Health, and gay men and women in New York still kiss Koch's ass, as gay men and women still think Ronald Reagan is peachy wonderful, and gay people in Massachusetts think that Ted Kennedy is wonderful, and he is in charge of health issues in the Senate and he has been silent and cowardly about AIDS for six long years, and how many dead brothers have to be piled up in a heap in front of your faces before you learn to fight back and scream and yell and demand and take some responsibility for your own lives?

I am telling you they are killing us and we are letting them!

Yes, I am screaming like an hysteric. I know that. I look and sound like an asshole. I told you this was going to be my last tirade and I am going to go out screaming so fucking rudely that you will hear this coarse, crude voice of mine in your nightmares. You are going to die and you are going to die very, very soon unless you get up off your fucking tushies and fight back!

Unless you do—you will forgive me—you deserve to die.

I never thought I would come to say anything like that. Nobody *deserves* to die.

I recently spoke at a *Village Voice* AIDS Forum in New York on a panel with Dr. Ron Grossman, who has one of the largest gay practices in New York. "Larry," he said to me, "our most outrageous early pronouncements are short of the mark. And so have been our efforts. We are so *behind.*"

AIDS is our holocaust. Tens of thousands of our precious men are dying. Soon it will be hundreds of thousands. AIDS is our holocaust and Reagan is our Hitler. New York City is our Auschwitz.

"Holocaust" is another word for "genocide."

"Genocide" is a word I hear myself and others using more and more frequently. You don't hear it as much as you hear words like "mandatory testing" or "no sex education in the schools" or "no condom ads on TV."

Why doesn't everybody realize that all the screaming and yelling going on about "education" and "mandatory testing" is one whale of a red herring?

Why doesn't everyone realize that while all the hatred and fury from the right wing, from the fundamentalists, Mormons, Southern Baptists, born-agains, Charismatics, Orthodox Jews, Hasidic Jews, Phyllis Schlafly, Paul Cameron, Governor Deukmejian, Representative Dannemeyer, Jesse Helms, Jerry Falwell—and all their equally as vocal supporters—goes on, that while they are screaming and yelling about the naughtiness of condoms and sex education and homosexuality, the killing culprit virus continues to spread and spread and spread and kill and kill and kill. While Rome burns, the Falwells fiddle, fanning their fundamentalists into fury against the faggots—and the junkies and the niggers and the spics and the whores and . . .

And they *know* it!

It is perfectly clear to me—no matter what Ronald Reagan and his henchmen say—that no substantial battle for a cure will be mounted while he is in office and that we must endure, at the least, another eighteen months of untended, *intended* death.

Very consciously they *know* that the more noise they can make, the more stalling tactics they can put into action, with the aid of their President, who supports them, and with the aid of his staff and his Cabinet and his Vice-President and his Attorney General and his Justice Department and his Supreme Court and his Secretary of Education and his various Secretaries and Assistant Secretaries of Health and Human Services and his director of the National Institutes of Health and his Centers for Disease Control—the more gays and blacks and Hispanics will die.

They *know* this! I believe it is a conscious act.

And we are allowing it!

We have fallen into their trap!

Our leaders—such as they are—their energies are consumed fighting these battles against mandatory testing and for better education—and no one is fighting the NIH for drugs and increased protocol testing and faster research. I am telling you that there are drugs and treatments out there that can prolong the quality of our lives and you are not getting them and no one is fighting for them and these drugs and treatments are caught up in so much red tape that they are strangled in the pipeline and the Reagan administration knows this, knows all this, and does nothing about untangling the red tape and half the gay men here can die because of it.

Yes, by our own passivity we are actively colluding with, and participating in, our own genocide.

We are allowing ourselves to be knocked off one by one. Half the gay men here could be dead in five years.

Our gay organizations are weak and *still* don't work with each other and our AIDS organizations have *all* been co-opted by the very systems they were formed to make accountable and you all sit by and allow it to happen when it's your lives that are going down the tubes.

Politicians understand only one thing: PRESSURE. You don't apply it—you don't get anything. Simple as that.

And it must be applied day by week by month by year. You simply can't let up for one single second. Or you don't get anything. Which is what is happening to us.

For six years I have been trying to get the gay world angry enough to exert this pressure. I have failed and I am ashamed of my failure. I blame myself—somehow I wasn't convincing enough or clever enough or cute enough to break through your denial or self-pity or death wish or self-destruction or whatever the fuck is going on. I'm very tired of trying to make you hear me.

I'm shutting up and going away. The vast majority of the gay world will not listen to what is so simple and plain. That there are so few voices as strident as mine around this country is our tragedy. That there is not one single gay leader who has any national recognition like Gloria Steinem or Cardinal O'Connor or Jerry Falwell or Jesse Jackson is also our tragedy. Why is that? Why does every gay spokesperson finally just collapse under the apathy of trying to make you listen—and failing, failing utterly.

Don't you ask yourselves quite often the Big Question: Why am I still alive? Untouched? At some point I did something the others did. How have I escaped?

Don't you think that obligates you to repay God or fate or whomever or whatever, if only your conscience, for this miraculous fact: I am still alive. I must put back something into this world for my own life, which is worth a tremendous amount. By not putting back, you are saying that your lives are worth shit, and that we deserve to die, and that the deaths of all our friends and lovers have amounted to nothing.

I can't believe that in your heart of hearts you feel this way. I can't believe you want to die.

Do you?

I guess this is the angriest speech I have ever delivered. I was pretty fed up and tired. Boston was an unlikely city to deliver it—they're a quiet, polite bunch up there, and the local gay papers had never been very kind to me. But this group kept calling me up, offering me a thousand bucks (I'd never been paid to speak before), and I decided I was going to diva-out and make my farewell appearance. And what better place than historic Faneuil Hall?

And for a while, I really meant it. Even though, much to my surprise, because as I'd harangued them they'd sat there stone-faced, I received a standing ovation; even though, much to my surprise, I got letters from as far away as France and places like Utah and Nevada, from strangers begging me not to quit. I'd had it.

I don't know why I can't confess to burnout when it happens to me, but I can't. I told everyone that I was quitting activism. I'd devote my energy to writing my plays and trying to get them on and writing another novel and trying again to get *The Normal Heart* made into a movie. You'll see, you'll see, I said. Larry's never going to make another speech again.

None of my friends believed me.

Whose Constitution Is It, Anyway?

I never knew what it felt like to be a nigger or a spic. Now I know. I'm a fag. Fags and niggers and spics aren't protected by the Constitution. Nor are junkies, whores, and broads.

Discrimination—consciously allowing some people to be treated as inferiors—is on the verge of totally bankrupting this country: financially, creatively, and morally.

This is not a good time in history to be a gay man or a lesbian, but particularly a gay man. I don't know if there ever was a completely good time to be gay, but for a little while there we were making some headway toward equality and acceptance. Until Ronald Reagan and AIDS came along, unfortunately at the same time.

I know you're celebrating the Constitution today. I don't feel very much like celebrating. The Constitution, as it is being administered today, doesn't protect me in the ways I need protection. In fact, I'm ashamed to be an American today—ashamed of how this precious document is being hypocritically

---

* Remarks made to a symposium sponsored by the New York Civil Liberties Union on Thursday, September 7, 1987, to celebrate the two-hundredth anniversary of the United States Constitution.

misread and misapplied to suit those who would wish me and all like me dead. I personally think that conscious genocide is going on. This administration's determination—which has persisted for a very long seven years—not to do anything sufficient to fight the AIDS epidemic can only be construed as an attempt to see that minority populations they do not favor will die. Seven years, 25,000 dead, over 50,000 cases, a quarter-million predicted in a few years' time, soon after that to be a million— and still there is no one in charge of combating AIDS, and still this city and this country do not provide adequate essential services, and still this government will not release the many life-saving drugs available in other countries, or educate the public so that a poor Florida family is not burned out of everything they have in this world.

I am going to tell you something you've never heard before. I am going to tell you that the AIDS pandemic is the fault of the white, middle-class, male majority. AIDS is here because the straight world would not grant equal rights to gay people. If we had been allowed to get married, to have legal rights, there would be no AIDS cannonballing through America.

The concept of making a virtue out of sexual freedom, i.e., promiscuity, to use that loaded word, came about because gay men had nothing to call their own *but* their sexuality. The heterosexual majority has for centuries denied us every possible right of human dignity that the Constitution was framed to provide to all. The right to marry. The right to own property jointly without fear that the law will disinherit the surviving partner. The right to hold a job as an openly gay person. The right to have children. The right not to be discriminated against in just about every area and avenue and byway and nook and cranny that can be found in which hatred is stored. Indeed—the right to walk down the street holding hands, as you do when you are freely in love. Yes, the right to love. We are denied the right to love. Can you imagine being denied the right to love?

So, rightly or wrongly—wrongly as it turned out—we decided we would make a virtue of the only thing you didn't have control over: our sexuality. Had we possessed these rights you denied us, had we been allowed to live respectably in a community as equals, there would never have been an AIDS. Had we been allowed to marry, we would not have felt the obligation to be promiscuous.

The poor, black, and Hispanic have also been forced into AIDS by your oppression. The awfulness of their destitution and deprivation, the absolutely zero chance they face to better their status in the world, forces them to seek peaceful respite and brief relief in the only oblivion available to them—the never-never land of drugs—which drugs, I might add, this country, for all the "Just Say No" mentality of an imbecilic First Lady, makes remarkably available through inept law enforcement and just plain looking the other way.

AIDS, having thus been caused to seed and sprout, is allowed to grow and fester and increase a millionfold. Yes, indeed, the white man made AIDS—the heterosexual white man. The heterosexual white man with money. The greedy heterosexual white man with money, who, two thousand years into the so-called Christian era, is still boss and master.

I am not going to speak in legalese, or cite the wretched decisions of the Supreme Court against us, or quote you lines from the Constitution or its Fourteenth Amendment or from the Bill of Rights. I am only going to say that some 25 million people constitute a sizable minority who are entitled to the same rights as everyone else. We do not practice behavior that can be changed, despite what that horrible monster, Robert Bork, or that equally horrible monster, the dogma of the Catholic Church, maintains as one reason for denying us these rights—that homosexuality can be changed. For decades, the psychiatric couches of the world sagged under the weight of gay people trying to change. At last, enlightened knowledge is finally beginning to concede the battle. We are born just as heterosexuals are born, just as people with blue eyes or people who are left-handed are born. Twenty-five million people cannot all be the result of any neurotic maladjustment or anything mothers or fathers do or don't do. Twenty-five million people are too many, too high a figure, to be anything but born, just as everyone else is born.

For our institutions—the Church, the Pope, the State, the Supreme Court—to pretend otherwise is, quite simply, immoral. How dare they presume to speak for God and for

Everyman? Because of these immoral institutions and their immoral pronouncements, we have been estranged from our families, and we have been forced to create a ghetto. We have been forced to suffer. We were forced into AIDS.

Would that 25 million people were not so frightened and not so invisible and had more courage to say out loud, all and at once: We are equal, whether you like it or not.

But we are frightened of you, with good reason, because of what you have done to us and continue to do to us, which is yet another tragedy, this fear of ours. I do not think the Constitution had fear, as well as enforced suffering, in mind as a prerequisite for minorities living under it. But so it has turned out.

I have learned, during these past seven years, to hate. I hate everyone who is higher in the pecking order and in being so placed, like some incontinent pigeon, shits all over all of those below. And, sadly, tragically, as more and more of my friends die—the number is way over two hundred by now—I hate this country I once loved so much. And as each day Ronald Reagan and the Catholic Church and various self-styled spokespeople for God—the Right Wing, the Moral Majority, fundamentalists, Mormons, Southern Baptists, born-agains, Orthodox Jews, Hasidic Jews, La Rouchies, Jesse Helms, Representative Dannemeyer, Governor Deukmejian, Phyllis Schlafly, Jerry Falwell, enemies all—take the law into their own hands, a law that neither the framers of the Constitution nor Christ himself, if indeed there ever was a Christ, ever envisioned would be so used to cause the deaths of fellow men, I not only hate, but I know there will never be freedom, or peace on earth, or America the Beautiful, or Oh, Beautiful for Spacious Skies.

Oh, say, can you see? our national anthem asks. Yes, I can see. I see a country more and more divided by hate. I see a country where the rich ignore the poor. I see a country where selfishness exceeds all other character traits. I see a country where education is no longer valued as the necessary force to give us strength and knowledge and compassion. I see a country where the media is controlled by and prepared for the privileged. I see a country where those less privileged have a voice that diminishes day by day until our cries are only heard as whispers. I see a country—and, I might add, a city—where crime and corruption and political chicanery and thefts of every conceivable sort are such a daily occurrence that we no longer protest and can no longer imagine a world otherwise. I see a country that the framers of the Constitution would be ashamed of. I know I am.

My country 'tis of thee? Oh, beautiful for spacious skies? God bless America? Oh, say, can you see by the dawn's early light? Our hymns have all turned into horseshit.

So go ahead and celebrate the anniversary of this once-precious document. I cannot do so.

The audience for this symposium appeared to be composed mostly of elderly men and women, with nothing else to do, who filled their days attending activities like this one, costing nothing. The first time the word "gay" was mentioned, a number of them got up and walked out. While I spoke, I saw only stony faces and icy stares. When I finished the applause was scattered. When questions were asked for, a handsome and well-dressed elderly woman stood up and told me, with a huge, positive smile, and a forceful, positive tone in her voice, that I must not talk about black people the way I had done, that it was possible for all people with the right attitude to improve their lot and better their lives, that she had seen, during her lifetime, the huge amount of progress in the black community, and that she thanked the Lord God for this and knew that He would carry on doing such a Fine Job for black people everywhere, everyone, every day.

Before the President's Commission

I'm a cofounder of Gay Men's Health Crisis, this country's first and largest community self-help AIDS organization, and founder of ACT UP—the AIDS Coalition To Unleash Power, a gay and straight group that's picketed, among others, the White House, *The Saturday Evening Post*, St. Patrick's Cathedral, and is at this moment picketing outside this meeting itself.

The fastest way this horrible epidemic can be stopped is to find a cure. Dr. Burton Lee, of your Commission, has been quoted as saying that you will not concern yourself with the basic science of AIDS. But the field of AIDS research is a huge mess. It's strangled in bureaucratic red tape, inefficiency, and a lack of cooperation among people, agencies, and countries.

We fought so hard for money. Congress has finally appropriated money. Now we find this money is either not being spent at all—hard as that may be to believe—or is being spent foolishly. The system set up by Dr. Anthony Fauci of NIH, of designated hospitals called ATEUs—AIDS Treatment Evaluation Units—is still, *after two years*, not functioning tolerably.

* Testimony before Hearings of the Presidential AIDS Commission, Washington, D.C., September 9, 1987.

Money for testing twelve thousand patients with promising drugs has been available for over a year. As of July, less than one thousand of these slots were filled. AZT—already approved by the FDA and effective for only half of those taking it—is still the main drug being tested. Other promising treatments are ignored. Dr. Fauci—who's been described by many AIDS experts as "in way over his head"—takes up to two years to make decisions that an organization like the American Foundation for AIDS Research can make in three months. The situation at NIH is now so bad that some drug companies and hospitals would prefer not to work with them at all. Couldn't some system be devised by which more *direct* funding is available, bypassing the NIH quagmire? Why must NIH get *all* the money? We in New York think we've found such a way. We've set up our own Community Research Initiative, with its own Institutional Review Board. The manufacturers of Ampligen—tired of waiting for NIH—are so excited about our CRI they're preparing a $4-million protocol. We'll provide two hundred patients—they'll provide this most promising drug, personnel, and money.

From the very beginning, we in the gay community have begged to do such as this. Let us help! Let us be your guinea pigs. You must remember that time is not on our side. Rules and laws that were formulated for slower fatal illnesses, or accidents such as those from thalidomide, simply don't apply with AIDS when patients have only two years to live, and something infectious is going around.

Our desperate circumstances often make us better informed than most doctors. Our grapevine often tells us about effective new treatments first. We pass this information to NIH and we're ignored. Anecdotal evidence is dismissed with holier-than-thou hauteur. AL 721 remains largely untested, even after a glowing report two years ago in the *New England Journal of Medicine*, as does Colony Stimulating Factors, which received similar praise. We've now learned, by sheer accident, that antabuse—the harmless medication given to help alcoholics—has an ability to raise T-cells. Antabuse, it turns out, is made up of the same molecules as Imuthiol. We've been begging for the testing of Imuthiol for a year. Why is there no mechanism available to *immediately* begin pilot studies with harmless antabuse? Must we wait two years while Dr. Meyers at NIH develops her protocols and Dr. Fauci's drug-selection committee has meeting after meeting, only to arrive—as they often do because they are so big and unwieldy and so timid—at no conclusion.

The FDA is a *passive* organization; you must go to them and prove everything *to* them. But often valuable drugs are controlled by inexperienced, poor, or inept companies that don't know how to maneuver the treacherous FDA waters. Why is there no mechanism in place to *actively* help these companies?

Now we face the growing difficulty of finding and keeping experienced personnel. The head of New York's Mt. Sinai ATEU gave as his excuse for his abysmal record that he couldn't find doctors or nurses willing to work on AIDS. NYU can't find data-base *computer operators* who aren't frightened. Soon we're going to find that not only is all the money there, the drugs and patients ready—but there's no staff to administer.

Indeed, the best scientists and researchers seem to be too scared to come anywhere near AIDS at all. Thus we're at the mercy of Drs. Broder and Gallo of NIH, who use their positions of power to intimidate. Indeed, Gallo is known at NIH as "the Godfather."

We implore you to investigate these areas. The epidemic will be in its *eighth* year by the time you report. Yet another precious year lost! The federal government's own General Accounting Office has proclaimed that there is a "perceived lack of leadership which is preventing a quick response."

You begin with many strikes against you in the eyes of the world. Much has appeared in the media about your credibility— and the fact that a *majority* of your membership is *on record* as saying something offensive about gay people. Right now, we don't expect you to either accomplish much or put aside your personal prejudices. Quite frankly, we think many of you would as soon see us dead.

But sometimes the challenge makes the man or woman. There are many instances in history where the most unlikely heroes have emerged and triumphed over their perceived images. We pray this will be one of those rare and precious and God-inspired occasions.

In closing, I would like to remind you of a few gay people who are a part of your history, too. Leonardo da Vinci, who painted *The Last Supper.* Michelangelo, who painted the Sistine Chapel and sculpted the most beloved *Pietà.* King James I, who undertook the most famous translation of the Bible. St. Augustine. Cardinal Newman. Cardinal Spellman. Pope Julius II. Pope Paul VI. Pope Benedict IX. Pope Sixtus IV. Pope John XXII. Pope Alexander VI. Pope Julius III. Joan of Arc.

Thank you.

I delivered this list while staring Cardinal O'Connor right in the eye.

Oh, My People

In reading over my collected diatribes of the past years, I realized I still am unable to resolve this fundamental problem—how to inspire you without punishing you.

We must live with facts that become more horrible with every passing minute. And no sooner do we fight one engagement than another one pops up in yet a completely different theatre of war. And we are losing to AIDS, at a rate that accelerates with every single minute.

I know we are all so tired of mourning. Because, as Mart Crowley said in *Boys in the Band*, "it takes a fairy to make something pretty"—we have managed to turn mourning into some kind of art form. I simply cannot attend another funeral or memorial service, although I know I shall. I often think I don't have any tears left.

I turned on the TV last night, and there, on "ABC World News Tonight," the Person of the Week was our own Cleve

* Acceptance speech delivered upon receiving the Arts and Communication Award at the Sixth Annual Human Rights Campaign Fund Dinner, Grand Ballroom, Waldorf Astoria, October 17, 1987.

Jones and there was that quilt—*that quilt!*—and I started crying again. And I couldn't stop crying.

I pray so much that our magnificent March on Washington is a mandate for us all. I pray it's a beginning, and not a last dying gasp, because we're so exhausted. Will every man and woman who danced down the middle of Pennsylvania Avenue return home to reinforce that energy and commitment in their lives and to their friends and families and jobs? Or was it, for them, just a dance down the middle of the road?

But what happened in Washington was, as Nelson Mandela would say, just another link in a long, long struggle.

They didn't give us very much time to feel good. This past week, after our return, came the Jesse Helms hate bill. Ninety-four senators voted *for* that bill. With the exception of Senators Weicker and, surprisingly, Moynihan, every single friend we thought we had suddenly turned against us. Then came the Dannemeyer hate bill. It's almost as if we're being immediately punished for our March. Slap them down quickly before they get too uppity. Even though the stingy media coverage robbed us, once again, of the accurate report of our true numbers, Washington saw that 650,000 of us were there, and now they're going to show us how powerful they are.

I'm afraid.

I've never said that out loud to you before. I think the torrents of hate are really just beginning. I don't think we've begun to see the horrors of what they're going to do to us. And we're crying "Genocide" now.

Oh, my people, I beg you to hear me. We are woefully unprepared:

We still have no leaders with national recognition.

We still have not learned how to broker our power.

We still don't know how to deliver votes in blocks to politicians.

We still have no national publication that is worthy of respect.

We still have no national organizations that are strong.

We have many small organizations that don't cooperate, many duplicating the same efforts and budgets and responsibilities and fighting for the same turf. We have too many Boards

of Directors and Task Forces and Defense Funds and Advocates and Action Councils and AIDS Networks and Coalitions
and Alliances for this and that. Each fights for the same dollars
and, hence, none of them receives enough to be truly effective.
The AMA has over 100 lobbyists. The tobacco industry has over
250. Twenty-five million gay people have—five.

The time has come when we must consolidate. We need one
or two powerhouse organizations, as blacks and women and
Jews have learned. Numbers, numbers, numbers, that's what
scares them, numbers, and we have to ram our numbers down
their fucking throats!

In my writing, I make a lot of comparisons between gays
now and the Jewish community before the war. The Jews
thought of themselves as good Germans first and good Jews
second. When the horror started, they couldn't believe what
their own fellow Germans were doing to them.

After the war, the Jewish leaders, those who were still alive,
came together in one room and determined that what had happened must never happen again. They vowed they would speak
with only one voice, and they would keep their arguments in the
confines of that one room, and the world would never see their
divisiveness in public again. And they've pretty much operated
successfully in that fashion ever since.

Somehow we've got to sit down in one room. From across
the nation, we've got to summon our boards of directors and
our executive directors and our rich and powerful. Our prominent professionals. Our well-connected. Our closeted presidents
of corporations and banks and the partners in law and accounting firms. In this room alone tonight is an assortment of talent,
brains, and money that should be enough to move mountains.

We are prioritizing our battles in the wrong order. There is
only one thing that is going to save us. The battle is, first and
foremost, for a cure. And we're not fighting this battle.

Definitive studies in San Francisco now prove beyond any
doubt that after six and a half years, 76 percent of those with
the virus will definitely come down with ARC or AIDS if they
have no treatment at all. This percentage gradually increases
in the following years to almost 100 percent. Even if my current
candidate for Public Enemy Number One, Dr. Anthony Fauci

of NIH, were to be on top of the situation today, 76 percent of those with the virus would still come down with ARC or AIDS.

We all now know there are many potentially life-saving drugs, almost all of which are available somewhere else in the world, that are simply not being tested here with speed and urgency, and there is not one single humanitarian reason why they aren't available to us. We all know the system of treatment centers that Fauci has set up isn't working. We know he's been given $141,349,398 to use for testing promising new drugs and that he's had this money for two years and five months and *still* he isn't spending it or testing anything much beyond AZT, which half of all AIDS patients cannot tolerate. So half of all AIDS patients are being told to just lie down and die. And AZT only works for about eighteen months. I've seen the list of all NIH protocols planned for the next five years. Eighty-seven percent of these are still for AZT. Not one of the drugs we've been begging for for three years is on this list. Until these are tested, how dare NIH tell us what won't work! We know the NIH receives $8.2 billion each and every year.

We are being murdered.

Oh, my people, why don't you hear me when I use this word "murdered?" Why don't you believe me when I tell you that Dr. Fauci and his boss, Dr. Wyngaarden, and our President, Ronald Reagan, and our mayor, Edward I. Koch—all megalomaniacs playing God—are murdering us?

When even one of our enemies, Cardinal O'Connor, starts talking about the need for a Manhattan Project to deal with AIDS—as he did on Thursday—is this not impetus enough at last for our leaders to meet in one room and consolidate our power toward demanding the very same and mobilizing all our energies to bringing such a Manhattan Project about?

I want to tell you about the Community Research Initiative: CRI. This is an offshoot of the PWA Coalition that is desperately seeking endowment. Its intention is to test drugs directly on patients in our own community, bypassing all government red tape. Results would be faster, cheaper, and we'd know very quickly if these drugs were working. Easily half of all gay men in San Francisco and New York are now infected with the virus. We are told *half of all gay men in San Francisco and New*

York are now infected with the virus! We are walking time
bombs. We have guns to our heads. Seventy-six percent of
those of us infected will come down with ARC or AIDS if we
receive no treatment at all. Latest CDC figures are worse than
ever: 95 to 98 percent of patients die within three years. We
simply can't wait for Dr. Fauci or Ronald Reagan or Edward
Koch. We can't wait for HRA and HHS and FDA and CDC and
PHS and NIH, the alphabet soup that is our government. Ron-
nie is senile and Nancy now is sick and cabinet members and
top officials are now resigning in droves and we face fifteen
more months of a sinking ship and we can't sink with it, we
must act! A number of prominent New York doctors are connected with CRI: Dr. Donald Armstrong of Sloan-Kettering,
Dr. Joseph Sonnabend, and our devoted friend and ally, Dr.
Mathilde Krim. We must fund CRI and put it into operation as
swiftly as is humanly possible. I beg you to be generous to it.
We must, repeat, *must* make the CRI work. Tom Hannan and
Michael Callen are here tonight, should any of you want to give
them checks or ask questions. Tom and Michael—stand up so
we can see two men of courage and vision.

I find it upsetting that the American Foundation for AIDS
Research, which CRI begged for funds, refused them, despite
appeals from Dr. Krim. Quite frankly, the less the wonderful
Dr. Krim is allowed to speak for AmFar, the less I like AmFar.
Slowly, she appears to be becoming a victim of and silenced by
a board of directors composed of many NIH monsters, or doctors funded by NIH monsters, so that AmFar, which is now
receiving millions and millions of dollars in charitable contributions, is unable to pressure the very NIH, which is not doing the
job it should be doing in the first place. Oh, the nooses tighten
and strangle us all to death.

I am ashamed of AmFar, as I now begin, once again, to
become proud of GMHC. Under Nathan Kolodner, GMHC is
moving forward in directions so many of us have begged it to
take for so long. But GMHC cannot take care of the world,
which is what it is being asked to do.

With pride, I close by acknowledging ACT UP. The AIDS
Coalition to Unleash Power—now almost one thousand very
energetic men and women who glory in nothing more than
protesting in the streets. I cannot tell you how infinitely moving

this organization is—this new generation that has no political agenda other than fighting against AIDS—many of them young men who never knew gay life free from fear, a life that I and many of you were, oh, so privileged to know. Their commitment is astounding. They have picketed and yelled and screamed and been arrested on some dozens of occasions—outside the White House, before the President's AIDS Commission, they totally destroyed Pat Robertson's presidential launch—and we will protest this coming Monday at twelve-thirty at City Hall at an AIDS Conference of Mayors and on Tuesday from three to seven at the United Nations, at their emergency plenary session on AIDS. I beg all of you to come and join us at both of these and at our Monday-night meetings at seven-thirty at the Community Center.

In a desperate struggle to secure their new homeland, the Jewish people in Palestine fighting to establish Israel had an organization called the Irgun. It was an underground guerrilla army, and its members were extremely disciplined and daring. They started fires. They threw bombs. They kidnapped. They assassinated. They executed their enemies. They won. Dr. Mathilde Krim belonged to the Irgun. So did Dr. Ruth.

We are such passive people, we gay people. We take all the shit they lay on us and then we lie down and take some more. And then we lie down some more and take even more. And more and more and more and more and more.

Oh, my people, I beg you to listen to me. I say all of this because I love you and I don't want to leave you or lose you.

And I thank the Human Rights Campaign Fund very much for my Arts and Communication award.

The award was presented to me by Nathan Kolodner, the president of GMHC. It was his idea to do so. It was the first time in four years that a public gesture of reconciliation was made by GMHC, and we hugged each other.

I was able, at the beginning of my remarks, to acknowledge my brother and sister-in-law, Arthur and
Alice Kramer, Joseph Papp and his wife, Gail Merrifield,
and Dr. Lawrence Mass, the only cofounder of GMHC
still living, along with me, in America (Ed White is in
Paris; Paul and Paul and Nathan are dead)—all of whom
were in the audience. I was particularly happy to make
Larry stand up and hear the huge applause for him; he
is one of the true heroes of these years of horror; his
impeccable medical reporting during those first years
was the only information most of us had, and he has not
been remembered for it or honored for it nearly sufficiently.

A wise friend urged me not to be so over-rhetorical
in my choice of "Oh, My People" for my running refrain.
I guess it looks corny in print, but it sounded good in the
Waldorf. If it does seem too much (Wise Friend had
recommended "Oh, My Friends")—well, it won't be the
first time I've erred in that direction. Anyway, I like it.

An Open Letter to Dr. Anthony Fauci

I have been screaming at the National Institutes of Health since I first visited your Animal House of Horrors in 1984. I called you monsters then and I called you idiots in my play *The Normal Heart* and now I call you murderers.

You are responsible for supervising all government-funded AIDS-treatment research programs. In the name of right, you make decisions that cost the lives of others. I call the decisions you are making acts of murder.

At hearings on April 29th before Representative Ted Weiss (D.-N.Y.) and his House Subcommittee on Human Resources, after almost eight years of the worst epidemic in modern history, perhaps to be the worst in all history, you were pummeled into admitting publicly what some have been claiming since you took over some three years ago.

You have admitted that you are an incompetent idiot.

Over the past four years, $374 million has been allocated for AIDS treatment research. You were in charge of spending much of that money.

It doesn't take a genius to set up a nationwide network of

* *Village Voice*, May 31, 1988, and *San Francisco Examiner*, June 26, 1988.

testing sites, commence a small number of moderately sized treatment efficacy tests on a population desperate to participate in them, import any and all interesting drugs (now numbering approximately two hundred) from around the world for inclusion in these tests at these sites, and swiftly get into circulation anything that *remotely* passes muster. Yet, after three years, you have established only a system of waste, chaos, and uselessness.

It doesn't take a genius to announce that you have elected to personally supervise the study of a broad range of new drugs. Yet, two years later, you are forced to admit you've barely begun.

It doesn't take a genius to request, as you did, 126 new staff persons, receive only eleven, *and then keep your mouth shut about it.*

It takes an incompetent idiot!

To quote Representative Henry Waxman (D.-Calif.) at the above hearings: "Dr. Fauci, your own drug selection committee has named twenty-four drugs as high priority for development and trials. As best I can tell, eleven of these twenty-four are not in trials yet. Six of these drugs have been waiting for six months to more than a year. Why the delays? I understand the need to do what you call 'setting priorities' but it appears even with your own scientists' choices, the trials are not going on."

Your defense? "There are just confounding delays that no one can help. . . . We are responsible as investigators to make sure that in our zeal to go quickly, we do the clinical study correctly, that it's planned correctly and executed correctly, rather than just having the drug distributed. . . ."

Now you come bawling to Congress that you don't have enough staff, office space, lab space, secretaries, computer operators, lab technicians, file clerks, janitors, toilet paper; and that's why the drugs aren't being tested and the network of treatment centers isn't working and the drug protocols aren't in place. You expect us to buy this bullshit and feel sorry for you? YOU FUCKING SON OF A BITCH OF A DUMB IDIOT, YOU HAVE HAD $374 MILLION AND YOU EXPECT US TO BUY THIS GARBAGE BAG OF EXCUSES!

The gay community has been on your ass for three years.

For thirty-six agonizing months, you refused to go public with what was happening (correction: *not* happening), and because you wouldn't speak up until you were asked pointedly and under oath by a congressional committee, we lie down and die and our bodies pile up higher and higher in hospitals and homes and hospices and streets and doorways.

Meanwhile, drugs we have been *begging* that you test remain untested. The list of promising untested drugs is now so endless, and the pipeline is so clogged with NIH and FDA bureaucratic lies, that there is no Roto-Rooter service in this shitty country that will ever muck it out.

You whine to Congress that you are short of staff. You don't need staff to set up hospital treatment centers around the country. The hospitals are already there. They hire their own staff. They only need money. You have money. YOU HAVE 374 MILLION FUCKING DOLLARS, FOR CHRIST'S SAKE!

The gay community has, *for five years,* told the NIH what drugs to test because we know and hear first what is working on some of us somewhere. You couldn't care less about what we say. You won't answer our phone calls or letters, or listen to anyone in our stricken community. What tragic pomposity!

The gay community has consistently told you that unless you move quickly your studies will be worthless because we are already taking drugs into our bodies that in desperation we locate all over the world (who can wait for you?!!), and all your "scientific" protocols are stupidly based on utilizing guinea-pig bodies that are "clean." You wouldn't listen, and now you wonder why so few sign up for your meager assortment of "scientific" protocols, which make such rigid demands for "purity" that no one can fulfill them, unless they lie. And why should those who can obtain the drugs themselves take the chance of receiving a placebo in one of your "scientific" studies?

To quote Representative Waxman again: "Aerosolized pentamidine was named High Priority *fourteen* months ago and there are still no people in trials. Everyone is now taking bootleg versions. Will you ever be able to get enough volunteers for placebo studies when it is now in routine use?"

How many years ago did we tell you about aerosol pentamidine, Tony? That this stuff saves lives. And we discovered it ourselves. We came to you, bearing this great news on a silver platter as a gift, begging you: Can we get it officially tested, can we get it approved by you so that insurance companies and Medicaid will pay for it (as well as other drugs we beg you to test) as a routine treatment, and our patients going broke paying for medicine can get it cheaper? You monster.

"Assume that you have AIDS, and that you've had pneumonia once," Representative Nancy Pelosi (D.-Calif.) said. "You know that aerosolized pentamidine was evaluated by NIH as highly promising. . . . You know as of today that the delays in NIH trials . . . may not be solved this year. Would you wait for [an NIH] study?"

You replied: "I probably would go with what would be available to me, be it available in the street or what have you. . . ."

We tell you what the good drugs are, you don't test them, then YOU TELL US TO GET THEM ON THE STREETS! You continue to pass down word from On High that you don't like this drug or that drug—WHEN YOU HAVEN'T EVEN TESTED THEM! You pass down word from On High that you don't want "to endanger the life of the patient." THERE ARE MORE AIDS VICTIMS DEAD BECAUSE YOU DIDN'T TEST DRUGS ON THEM THAN BECAUSE YOU DID!

You've yet to test Imuthiol, AS 101, dextran sulfate, DHEA, Imreg-1, Erythropoietin—all drugs that Gay Men's Health Crisis considers top priority. You *do* like AZT, which consumes 80 percent of your studies, even though Dr. Barry Gingell, GMHC's medical director, now describes AZT as a "a cumulative poison . . . foisted on the public." Soon there will be more AIDS victims dead because you did test drugs on them—the wrong drugs.

ACT UP was formed over a year ago to get experimental drugs into the bodies of patients. For one year ACT UP has tried every kind of protest known to man (short of putting bombs in your toilet or flames up your Institute) to get some movement in this area. One year later, ACT UP is still screaming for the same drugs they begged and implored you and your world to release. One year of screaming, protesting, crying, cajoling, lobbying, threatening, imprecating, marching, testifying, hoping, wishing, praying has brought nothing. You don't listen. No one listens. No one has ears. Or hearts.

Whose ass are you covering, Tony? (Besides your own.) Is it the head of your Animal House, the invisible Dr. James Wyngaarden, director of the National Institutes of Health (and may a Democratic President get him out of office *fast*)? Is it Dr. Vincent Devita, head of the National Cancer Institute, another invisible murderer who lets you be his fallguy? Or Dr. Otis Bowen, secretary of the Department of Health and Human Services, no doubt the biggest murderer on this list; George Schultz and Caspar Weinberger would never take the constricting bullshit from the Office of Management and Budget that Bowen wallows in. All you "doctors" have, continuously, told the world that All Is Being Done That Can Be Done. Now you admit that isn't so.

WHY DID YOU KEEP QUIET FOR SO LONG?!

I don't know (though it wouldn't surprise me) if you kept quiet intentionally. I don't know (though it wouldn't surprise me) if you were ordered to keep quiet by Higher Ups Somewhere and you are a good lieutenant, like Adolf Eichmann.

I do know that anyone who knows what you have known for three years—that, to quote Representative Weiss, "the dimension of the shortfall is such that you can't possibly meet your needs," and, to quote *The New York Times* and their grossly incompetent AIDS reporter, Philip Boffey (whose articles read like recycled NIH press releases; who doesn't know how to get The Other Side of any story; who refuses to investigate anything he christens A Fact), "Official Blames Shortage of Staff for Delay in Testing AIDS Drugs"—I repeat, anyone who has known all this and denied it for the past three years is a murderer, not dissimilar to the "good Germans" who claimed they didn't know what was happening.

I will also tell you two things I have learned in the last few weeks. New York doctors are now seeing AIDS patients who are not testing HIV-positive during the course of their illness. What does that say about your AIDS test? What does that say about the safety of the nation's blood supply? What does that say to the millions of people who have been tested and think they're fine when in fact they could still be carriers? As more and more cases of AIDS appear, there are going to be more and more bizarre phenomena like this. Everything is not going to fit neatly into your little, simpleminded, HIV-only package.

The New York Blood Center is discovering AIDS happening in people with no known risk behavior (translated: white heterosexuals who've never had contact with drugs or engaged in homosexual acts). But their funding sources (translated: Centers for Disease Control; New York City Department of Health; New York State Department of Health; U.S. Department of Health and Human Services) are suddenly uninterested in funding research that provides this kind of information. So the New York Blood Center has discontinued cataloging these cases. So the world can go on thinking AIDS only happens to gays, blacks, Hispanics, and junkies.

But then, I guess this kind of information is really not your problem. Your problem is to learn how to spend your own $374 million.

With each day I realize a little more that the gay community has lost the battle. And that we haven't even begun to experience the horrors that still await us—horrors even worse than those you represent. We have lost. No one important enough has ears. Or hearts.

You care, I'm told (although I no longer believe it). I've even heard you called a saint. You are in essence a scientist who's expected to be Lee Iacocca. But saints, miracle workers, good administrators, and brilliant scientists have imaginations vivid enough to know how to spend $374 million in a time of dire emergency. You have no imagination. You are banal (a word used so accurately to describe Eichmann).

Do I want you to leave? (Yes.) Could your replacement be more pea-brained than you? (Yes, it is possible.) Will this raving do any good at all? Will it make Congress shape you up? Will it make my own community's bureaucratically mired AIDS organizations finally ask the right questions? (Judy Peabody of GMHC, please take note.) Will Dr. Mathilde Krim ever—as she indicated she would—get the American Foundation for AIDS Research to fund the desperately needed and desperately needy Community Research Initiative, which is valiantly attempting to do what you should be doing, so tired are we of waiting for you to do it. (Leonard Bernstein and Harry Kraut, please take note.)

I have no answer to most of these questions. You may (God help us all) be the best that will be given us. You may, like John Erlichman, once accused, desire redemption and forgiveness by rethinking, retooling, and, like Avis, trying harder. Even more miraculous, those Supreme Murderers in the White House might tomorrow acknowledge that families simply everywhere have gay sons and daughters.

But I fear these are only pipe dreams and you'll continue to carry on with your spare equipment. The cries of genocide from this Cassandra will continue to remain unheard. And my noble but enfeebled community of the weak, the dying, and the dead will continue to grow and grow—until we are diminished.

I he level of rhetoric gets higher, the pitch more shrill. The separation between gay readers of this diatribe, for whom it reads with the utmost sane clarity, and straight readers, who think I've now gone round the bend, increases.

How do you finally get the system to work? How do you get important people to listen? And act?

After seven years, I no longer know.

I remember, while writing my earliest pieces, thinking they sounded very angry indeed. Rereading them now, they seem almost calm. Will this attack on Fauci, in a few years' time, sound calm? I think so.

After we had attacked each other in print for several years, it was gratifying that Richard Goldstein, the openly gay editor of the *Village Voice*, welcomed this piece into that publication, whose record on AIDS reporting, while better, is still pretty awful. But it's a strange publication—purchased, I think, mostly by yuppies who want the *Voice*'s encyclopedic listings of weekly Village events, and edited, for the most part, by heterosexual left-wing liberals, who have never been gays' best friends.

Indeed, where have been the voices of Norman Mailer, Saul Bellow, Irving Howe, Alfred Kazin, George Steiner, Victor Navasky, Philip Roth, Arthur Miller, Michael Harrington, Naomi Bliven—to name only a few I used to admire but have yet to hear from on the most crucial issue now facing modern man?

Dear Max

16 June 88

Mr. Max Frankel
The New York Times
229 West 43rd Street
New York, NY 10036

Dear Mr. Frankel,

Thank you very much for your letter of 8 June. I am pleased you thought my *Voice* "polemic" "brilliant." It's been picked up by about twenty newspapers across the country.

I feel your letter requires an answer, and a long one. You say that you "reject the paranoid theories about our suppression of news and I'm satisfied that after a slow start we're doing quite well on the AIDS story."

I must somehow prove to you that my "theories" about your "suppression of news" are not "paranoid" and that, indeed, the *Times* is still not doing a very good job of covering AIDS.

I thought the best way I might accomplish this was by simply taking your recent AIDS articles, day by day, and pointing out to you some facts about them.

■ ■ ■

Friday, June 3, page 1: Philip Boffey's lead article on Admiral
James Watkins and his Presidential AIDS Commission Report.
Boffey focuses almost exclusively on the report's antidiscrimination recommendation. For a report of many hundreds of
pages, containing 578 other recommendations, seven-eighths of
Boffey's prose is about one point only. Nowhere in the entire
article, or in the excerpts from the report itself you chose to
run, is any of its biting criticism of the FDA and NIH for their
tragic intransigence. So far as I can see, you were the only
major American newspaper to overlook this. As far as coping
with AIDS is concerned, there is no more important subject
today than getting experimental drugs into research protocols.
This is the one subject that the *Times* has been exceedingly bad
on, and, as you know, it's the one subject I feel is the most
important subject out there. Research.

[I had written Frankel on May 29th: "Boffey's articles read
like recycled press releases from NIH, or pharmaceutical companies, or various government agencies. He rarely bothers to
get the other side of any story, or opinions from dissenters. And
when he does, the way he uses them, writes them in, so obviously conveys his bias that these dissenters appear as crazies.
Well, as happens so often in science, in discovery, in anything
on the cutting edge, I submit to you that it is often the crazies
who make the discoveries. NIH, NCI, NIAID—none of these
has such a hot record on major cancer stuff."]

■ ■ ■

Sunday, June 5, page 1: Gina Kolata's article on the ability of
"the AIDS virus" to remain undetected. This story, about macrophages, is one year old. Macrophages have been written
about in the gay press for fully one year. Indeed, when I saw
Boffey at the Presidential Commission's meeting on September
9th, 1987, I asked him why he wasn't writing this story. He
knew nothing about it and didn't seem particularly interested
in finding out anything further. I offered him names of New
York doctors who were noting patients with AIDS testing negative for "the AIDS virus" over a long period of time.

[In my earlier letter, I'd said: "Boffey isn't the only one. Gina

Kolata, who wrote so well when she was at *Science* magazine, now appears to write most vapidly—her heart just doesn't seem to be in it, and a number of her stories appear to go against the grain of what she in fact thinks."]

■ ■ ■

Sunday, June 5, editorial: Nick Wade (if he indeed wrote this) has, in general, been one of your most effective observers of AIDS. He is accessible to outsiders, which Boffey, Kolata, and Dr. Lawrence Altman are not. This particular editorial is fine, but, again, there is absolutely no mention of Watkins's steaming criticism of FDA and NIH.

■ ■ ■

Thursday, June 9, page A-32: Boffey's article on the *Nature* magazine report warning on heterosexual spread. Why is this buried at the bottom of the back page? This is one of the most important issues today, and an extremely respectable magazine is saying something terrifying, and you not only bury it on the back page, but everything in Boffey's contorted prose is geared to refuting the *Nature* warning, calming the waters. Surely this article should have been on page one, and should have been longer and filled with fewer caveats, and Boffey should have sought supporting opinions from other experts who feel the same.

■ ■ ■

Monday, June 13, page A-13: Lawrence Altman's first report from the International AIDS Conference in Stockholm. I don't know what conference you sent this man to cover, but he's not at the same conference as reporters from the *Washington Post*, the *San Francisco Chronicle*, and the *Los Angeles Times*. Each report Altman has filed deals with only one issue. Every other reporter has filed stories containing four, five, or six major announcements. "AIDS outlook bleak." "Aren't we fortunate AIDS wasn't called GRID?" What kind of stupid article is this? Filled with filler, verbiage that doesn't say anything. On this day, Dr. Jonathan Mann of the World Health Organization presented frightening and comprehensive *detailed* figures and projections that even every major network

excerpted on the national evening news. Dr. Robert Gallo made
some specific predictions about vaccines, including the astonishing statement that there might never even be one that was any
good.

■ ■ ■

Tuesday, June 14, page B-4: Bruce Lambert's article on New
York State medical societies seeking to force State Health Department officials to deal with AIDS as a communicable disease.
There are two huge holes left open in this article. One is that
nowhere is mentioned any statement to refute the medical societies' spokesmen, to the effect that "the AIDS test" as presently available is not sufficiently useful a tool to do what the
societies want. The other is that you simply cannot use a statement like "He accused the state of bowing to homosexuals,"
without getting a statement from a homosexual source to balance it. And, boy, I wish we were that powerful in reality! I hear
so many remarks about "the tough tactics of gay lobbyists,"
which is just absurd. We have, in total, six full-time lobbyists
working for AIDS and are they not tough! To Bruce's credit, he
is your only reporter who, quite rightly, qualifies the putative
cause by saying "the virus believed to cause AIDS." Everyone
else has bought HIV hook, line, and sinker. There simply is no
agreement that HIV is the *only* cause.

[In my May 29th letter to Frankel, I'd written: "Bruce Lambert took me out to dinner to pick my brains. I thought this was
very enterprising of him, and I liked him, not only for that. I
gave him—it must have been a dozen or more story ideas, which
he wrote down greedily. I've called him several times since to
pass on a few more. Not one of these ideas has ever made it into
a story in the *Times*. When I asked him why, he said they'd all
been submitted, but had not been approved by those Higher
Ups to whom these decisions evidently fall." I've since learned
that all *Times* AIDS reporting falls under one of three desks:
Metro (for New York), National, and Science. Each desk has
one or two or three editors. Often AIDS stories aren't clearly
local or national or scientific: They're all three, or two of them.
Then, evidently, rivalries take over, disputes over turf, or the
story falls, by default, to the editor least interested in it, or a
story that contains political implications is handed to Science,

where all the nonscientific matter is edited out. The *Times*—and why should anyone be surprised—is as bureaucratically mired and inefficient as every other AIDS service provider. And if the story should be for the Sunday *Times,* or for "The Week in Review," or the magazine section, then there are yet *further* editors involved in the tussle.]

■ ■ ■

Tuesday, June 14, page B-4: Altman from Stockholm again. On the day when vital new evidence was presented about additional possibly causative viruses, Altman chooses to report on results of the experimental drug Imreg. Fine. As far as it goes. Nowhere does he mention that we have known about these results for about six months, that we have been clamoring for Imreg for over a year. Nowhere does he raise the troubling question: Why were the Imreg studies so small, when it has been known to be so promising for so long? He mentions that the company that produces it is "small." He doesn't tell us how hard it is for "small" companies to get cooperation from the FDA. He includes the most pathetic quote from "a spokesman from the Federal Food and Drug Administration," to whit, "We look forward to receiving the clinical data that would substantiate the claims being made for this drug." This breaks my heart. Neither *The New York Times* nor any other paper, except *The Wall Street Journal,* has done an exposé of the subtext of this FDA spokesman's response: The FDA is a *passive* organization. You have to present everything *to* them. Nowhere in this entire government is there any mechanism for *actively* helping a "small" company that doesn't have the savvy skills of a Burroughs Wellcome, the manufacturers of AZT, in maneuvering through the treacherous FDA (and NIH) waters. Here comes a promising drug, Imreg; why isn't the FDA spokesperson saying, "We look forward to doing everything in our power to helping Imreg gain approval and get out into the world." I beg of you—please get someone to write about the FDA not working at all, as Watkins's report so bravely pointed out.

■ ■ ■

Wednesday, June 15, page A-21: Altman, still from Stockholm, writing about the great efficacy of aerosol pentamidine. This story, too, is over one year old. Dr. Donald Armstrong at Sloan-Kettering ran his original study over a year ago, and the results of this study are widely known (not, certainly, from the *Times*), so much so that this drug is in widespread and general use just about everywhere in the world. I and many others have tried innumerable times to get various *Times* reporters (not Altman, who doesn't return phone calls, and has behaved like this since 1981) to write about this over this past year. No one was interested. Altman writes: "The National Institutes of Health is now sponsoring a large trial that is being conducted in several hospitals." This is a huge distortion of reality. You read my *Voice* "polemic." In it I quoted testimony from the Ted Weiss hearing in which Fauci was raked over the coals for *not* testing aerosol pentamidine a long time ago, and Fauci admitted that the trials were planned but still in the future, and that he, under pressure, admitted that if he had *Pneumocystis*, he'd go out in the streets to get this drug.

In this same issue of the *Times* there is an important letter to the editor from Arthur Leonard, a professor of law and an exceptionally able writer about AIDS legal concerns, in which he also takes issue with Philip Boffey for omitting vital facts from his June 3, page-one article on Admiral Watkins's recommendations—the heinous tactics Representative William Dannemeyer and Senator Jesse Helms have used to kill any possible legislative vehicle for achieving the protection against discrimination that the Watkins report makes top priority. How could you not be writing about these two murderous dumbbells?

■ ■ ■

Thursday, June 16, page A-25: My least favorite (edging out Boffey by a nose), Altman, again from Stockholm, reporting on the slowdown of AIDS in the addict population. (Would that it were so!) He must have gone home early. On this day, exceedingly important information was presented concerning the promising efficacy of *four* experimental treatments, including dextran sulfate and naltrexone. Indeed, the naltrexone results were reported by a New York doctor, Dr. Bernard Bihari, of SUNY-Brooklyn. Additionally, there was a vitally important report on the promising CD-4 (even the networks reported on this one), as well as promising reports from Israel on AL 721, and mixed results on Peptide-T. The *San Francisco Chronicle* ran *four* separate articles about AIDS and about this conference on this date. (The *Times*'s coverage of the entire conference, which was a very important conference, has been so sparse and piddling as to be tragic. It is a sad commentary when all three networks—particularly George Straight on ABC—do a better job covering a major happening than *The New York Times.*)

Information about these drugs is information this city should and must have, and you are not reporting it. How dare you overlook this? People are desperate for this kind of news above all other.

And you think I am "paranoid" about your suppression of the news!

■ ■ ■

Now some further thoughts: Your reporters just write the same stories everyone else writes. Mostly, when something "new" is reported in a medical journal, they just rewrite it and put it out. That's not reporting. That's really just a form of plagiarism. It doesn't take much talent to rewrite a medical journal article. Most of them contain news, as I've shown above, that's old news anyway, which we knew about a long time ago, and, in many instances, tried to get your people to write about a long time ago. No one does much "reporting" up there. What are you paying them for? To thumb through the medical journals as soon as they arrive on their desks?

Dextran sulfate: This is a terrific story. I've told Boffey and Lambert, as have others. It comes from Japan. It seems to raise T-cells. Doctors in New York have been sending couriers over for about six months to get it. As soon as the FDA heard about this, they clamped down, made it illegal to import it into this country, so that it's now seized at the borders if you try to bring it in. Further, the FDA instructed Japan not to sell it to Americans. The Japanese therefore made it a prescription drug—it had been available there over the counter *for twenty years*, with no reported bad effects. So now AIDS sufferers can't get it. Why aren't you writing stories like this? It puts the FDA to shame. Talk to Dr. Barbara Starrett about the tests she's doing with dextran sulfate. She is, by the way, one of the "AIDS

Heroes" profiled in the current issue of *7 Days.* Here is a local
doctor, sick and tired of waiting for the NIH and FDA to study
and release promising drugs, who is doing the damned (and
expensive and tedious) testing on her own. With her own patients. With her own money. She sent her own lover, Ann Silver
(who is hearing-impaired), over to Japan to courier supplies
back. Why aren't you writing human-interest stories like this?
Barbara's story has certainly been pitched to your boys and
girls.

Every single drug or treatment that is promising and that
we can't get hold of has a story of chicanery or slipups of some
sort. Susan Spencer said on "CBS News" the other night that
there are now *two hundred* drugs that are promising, and that
aren't available here. That's awful. Where are your reporters?
Isn't this suppression of vital news? Am I paranoid? I can't tell
you how many times many of us have tried to get your reporters to write these stories.

The stupid (if it weren't so tragic) story behind the unavaila-
bility of AL 721, for instance. It comes from the Weizmann
Institute, certainly a distinguished place. They licensed the pat-
ent, it seems, not to one of the international drug companies
that were after it, but to one of the members of the Weizmann
Institute's American board, a New York attorney, Leslie Jacob-
son, whose nephew had a tiny drug company with little track
record or, as it turned out, experience or ability to manufacture
the stuff in sufficient quality or quantity to supply the NIH for
their planned protocols. That's a tragic story, Mr. Frankel. You
haven't written it. The *New England Journal of Medicine*
described AL 721 as promising and worthy of study *three years
ago!* And it still remains improperly tested. And here are reports from Stockholm that it's still promising, three years later.

One of the problems is that your reporters are very
haughty. They aren't interested in putting their ears to the
ground. They're only interested in listening to establishment
doctors, most of whom don't know very much about AIDS
treatments because these treatments aren't recognized by the
FDA or the NIH. Why don't your reporters listen to the gay
community, which knows more about what's going on than
most doctors? Dr. Barry Gingell, the medical director of
GMHC, is now so frustrated that he puts out a GMHC treat-

ment newsletter that prints all of the stuff you should be printing. If the power of the *Times* isn't available to get the system to move forward on malfeasances, what good is the *Times* in a time of dire emergency?

Another story you refuse to track is the Community Research Initiative. This is an historic attempt by the gay community to test drugs on ourselves. Indeed, they did the aerosol pentamidine study with Dr. Armstrong of Sloan-Kettering, which, over a year ago, discovered the same thing that Altman is just now "reporting" from Stockholm. Your reporters are invited to all CRI press conferences, but they never show up. Dr. Mathilde Krim is on CRI's board. So is Dr. Armstrong. It is not a fly-by-night group. They desperately need media attention so they can raise money. They just got a small grant from Du Pont to test Ampligen—from Du Pont! A tiny community group that was sick and tired of waiting for NIH and FDA to test important drugs found, somehow, a way to legally set up their own protocols, and is doing invaluable work on a shoestring. Talk about a continuing human-interest story! But is the *Times* there? No.

Every time a black or Jewish group holds a protest or performs some act of civil disobedience, it's reported in the *Times*. Every time ACT UP protests, the *Times* never shows. This group of several thousand (which has even finally been profiled in *Newsweek*) has done monumental acts of civil disobedience in this town and in this country, and the *Times* never notices. They held a four-day, around-the-clock picketing of Sloan-Kettering last summer, and where were you? It's pretty hard to ignore a four-day, around-the-clock event, but you managed to do so. A very angry zap of Mayor Koch last week, which made the local TV news and the *Post* and the *Daily News*, but not the *Times*, prevented Koch from speaking for a full half hour, until he left in a huff. Why can't *our* activism be reported?

Did you know about the mess at the New York Blood Center? I tipped Bruce Lambert off to this many months ago. The *New York Observer* just ran a long article on part of the mess, but no one else has. It goes even further than they reported. Rather than be forced into admitting that a heterosexual rise is occurring in non-drug or non-gay-contact persons, which they are discovering, the Blood Center has discontinued tallying these results. That's a scandal! The *San Francisco Chronicle* ran an article yesterday on another aspect of this: "AIDS Suspected Behind Rise in Female Deaths." Evidently women diagnosed with other illnesses are now thought to have died from AIDS. Where are your reporters? I even think this one was on the wire service.

I could go on endlessly about other stories you're not reporting, or are reporting badly. I do hope you can concede that I've made a bit of a point in disputing your letter. I'd like to close with querying your last sentence. "Please don't make them [your reporters] hostile with unfounded and unsubstantiated accusations." (I hope I have more than substantiated my accusations!) I query your notion of what happens if and when my criticisms turn your folks hostile. Are you saying that criticism will turn them against writing about AIDS in a responsible fashion? (Not that they're doing so now.) That is what it *seems* you are saying. If that is so, and I can't believe you mean this, then your reporters are not any reporters I should like to have on the staff of any newspaper I want to read.

I hope you realize that I write this, and keep after you and yours, because, like so many others, I care deeply not only about AIDS, but about the *Times.* We all want it to be perfect, which nothing can be. But on AIDS, for some reason, you have been, from the very beginning, very poor indeed. Yes, you are better than you were under your hated and hateful predecessor, Abe Rosenthal. But you are just not yet good enough.

[I closed my May 29th letter with: "So, once again, after a short spurt of recovery, the *Times,* the supposed paper of record, has reverted to its earlier Rosenthalian blind lethargy. More and more books are being written about your awful showing—to go along with Randy Shilts's *And the Band Played On.* I have been interviewed for several of them, including ones written by academics, who seem to be very interested these days in the role, or lack of it, of proper media attention to the AIDS epidemic. No one has a very good word to say about the *Times,* before you or, really, during you."]

We have been writing to each other for so long that I feel we are somehow almost friends. Would it be permissible at this stage to deal with each other on a first-name basis?

I received a short note in return, which began with "Dear Larry" and was signed "Sincerely, Max," and which said, "Yes, first names help. So would more staff. Without agreeing on all your points, we would like to do yet more and are looking to find a way to get it done along with everything else."

I understand that both these letters of mine were circulated to all the desk editors and all the reporters I criticized. This both pleases me and surprises me, happily so. In the week following, Dr. Barry Gingell was taken out to lunch by Deputy Science Editor Erik Eckholm and reporter Gina Kolata, and asked to provide them with a list of important stories. *Times* metropolitan reporter Tom Morgan was assigned a feature article on ACT UP. Bruce Lambert was assigned to covering AIDS full time. And Washington AIDS reporter Philip Boffey is still there.

Max and I write to each other several times a month now. It's almost impossible for me to believe that the editor-in-chief of the world's most powerful newspaper actually answers my letters, and with occasional sympathy, but always politely and quickly. For the first six years of AIDS, the *Times* was edited by a monster. Abe Rosenthal would not only never respond to a letter, but he rarely allowed acknowledgment that gay people even existed. May he go down in history as the culpable villain he is. Along with his henchman, Dr. Lawrence Altman, the principal AIDS "reporter" for those long, silent years at the *Times.*

Max appears a kind man, certainly a liberal one. One of his first acts in office was to allow use of the word "gay" instead of "homosexual" as Rosenthal had demanded. But I don't think Max really comprehends that there are one million gay people in New York, and that a goodly number of us are his readers and his advertisers. His response to AIDS is that of a decent heterosexual responding to a few cries from the wilderness, rather than that of a pragmatic editor cognizant of the necessity that this million is entitled to have its history written about with the depth, frequency, and integrity granted to other minorities like blacks and Jews.

While most *Times* coverage has improved, the main AIDS reporter is still the incompetent Phil Boffey. I do not know what the specific problem with this man is. Is it a lack of compassion, a lack of energy, a lack of reportorial skills, or is he just plain dumb? Article after article finds him completely missing the main point of discussion. He always defers to the same few people for information or quotes of attribution. He does not understand AIDS, and yet he is the the principal *Times* spokesperson on it.

I think history will eventually record that it is one of the truly great tragedies—of an epidemic not lacking in them—that it fell to Altman and Boffey to be the principal AIDS investigators for *The New York Times*.

And so, I notice, I end as I began—with the *Times*. I suppose it's not a bad symbolic symmetry, the *Times*.

The times.

To relive these years, as I have done in preparing this book, has been to relive a lifetime. I've been plagued with mixed emotions: Dare I include this? Did I really write that? This makes me sound so self-serving. Or too self-righteous. Or too righteous, period. Or an ass. What a megalomaniac.

What are the main lessons I've learned? One is this: I no longer believe America is a country where one voice can make any difference.

I started out, in 1981, believing it could. Oh, I can see where certain things I raged against were now and then affected. But it shouldn't take so long when so many people are dying. And something infectious is going around. And everything's going to get much, *much* worse.

I also learned, after an earlier life of comparative privileges, what it's like not to have them anymore. I have learned—in a more tangible and visible way than I ever thought or was taught I would encounter in a "free" and "democratic" society—how gay people are hated and expendable.

I believe I said everything I said in the only way I knew how to say it at that moment. In so doing, I became the "activist" I never wanted to be. The angry kid I was found a way to use that anger. I'm no less angry now that I've grown up. But I'm much more tired.

Well, whatever I wrote, it's all here. The ups and downs of antagonisms and of friendships. The loss from death. The death of hope.

The making of an AIDS activist.

Part Two

Part Two

Report from the holocaust

I

I don't think any heterosexual can understand what it's like to be a homosexual man in New York today—or in any other major American city: Los Angeles, San Francisco, Houston, Dallas, Miami, Boston, Chicago, but particularly in New York, which, with some one million gay men and women, is the largest gay city in the world.

I don't understand much of it myself, and writing this essay has been yet another attempt to do just that. I've been asked, though rarely, by heterosexual friends: "How do you stand it? How do you live?" And I can't really answer, except to say something annoyingly clichéd like: "We all take it one day at a time," or, more often, "I try not to think about it," which is a lie but serves to cut off further discussion. It's not that I mind talking about it; it's just that I've come to find heterosexual inquiry just that, and only that: inquiry. More like checking to see what my opinion is of the latest movie. I've come to be very angry about this heterosexual attitude, and less tolerant of the perfectly valid (to them), reasonable excuses heterosexuals use to support it, as voiced by my brother, Arthur, a lawyer: "We have our own lives and our own set of problems; I don't ask you to fight my battles, don't expect and demand that I fight yours." So, rather than destroy what few straight friendships I have left, I've found myself changing the subject or, more often of late, withdrawing more and more from my straight friends and even my family.

Most gay men don't know how we're enduring it. If we're still healthy, we clutch that fact to our hearts and minds, and attempt to take strength from it: I am here, I am alive, I don't know *why* I'm alive, or how, but I am alive. I have never before, in my fifty-three years of living, been particularly grateful to be alive. It's just something I never thought about. It's a notion that always seemed to accompany facing old age and death. There'd always been good days and bad days then, mixed together.

I hesitate to state that over the past seven years I have lost some five hundred acquaintances and friends to AIDS. I realize that putting a figure to this loss is both gruesomely macabre and too Madison Avenue. It makes me sound weird: that I have for over seven years kept a record of these names. It also sounds vaguely opportunistic: trafficking in dead bodies to make a morbid point. Further, I think it makes me sound a bit—I don't know—self-serving? How could anyone *know* five hundred men? It sounds like I'm scouring to make a point, which, of course, I am. Nobody *knows* five hundred people, straight friends tell me disbelievingly, proving to me that this isn't the right approach for argument or pleas for help.

Because gays live in a ghetto, we know personally and generally recognize most of the people in it. We live together in this world-within-a-world: certain neighborhoods in Manhattan, Fire Island, the Hamptons; the discos we once danced in; the organizations we belong to, from religious congregations (gay synagogues, Catholic worship groups) to social ones like gay alumni from one's college, Men of All Colors Together, choruses and marching bands, to athletic teams: soccer and baseball and football (now even a Gay Games, which would be called the Gay Olympics, were it not for the Supreme Court disallowing it) to AA meetings, affiliations of gay physicians, social workers, men in advertising, the law, even the police, to

charitable endeavors, and, now, AIDS organizations in which
we attempt to take care of our own; or just walking down city
streets everywhere. But even in rural areas of New York
State and New Jersey and Staten Island, gays know where
other gays are. It's like the old American idea of life in a small
town. We know everybody.

We know who we are. When the first man who ever loved
me, a professor of mine at Yale, told me during my freshman
year in 1953 that, yes, we could all pretty much recognize each
other passing on the streets, I didn't believe him. How could one
tell? Well, one can mostly tell.

If an infectious illness were happening to Jews, in which
over 50 percent of their population was thought to be infected—one out of every two Jews—how many people would a
socially active Jew in, say, Rego Park, or Boro Park, or Wood-
mere, or Great Neck, or the upper West Side know? How many
Jews would a person like Cynthia Ozick or Laurence Tisch or
Bella Abzug or Edward Koch know? Such an occurrence would
seem devastating not only to their community, but to the world.
Happening to gay men, it doesn't seem to register very high on
the devastation scale. That's the problem.

Because I have helped to start two AIDS organizations, one,
Gay Men's Health Crisis, for self-help (though it was originally
founded to fight to make the world pay attention and help us)
and one, ACT UP—the AIDS Coalition to Unleash Power—for
political activism, and because I have written extensively about
the gay world, beginning with my novel, *Faggots*, which I
wrote between 1975 and 1978, and continuing with many pieces
of political journalism, I guess I know more gay people than
most, and more dead gay men than many. Too, because I am a
writer fascinated by everyone's story, I tend to recognize many
people who might not know me, but whom I know about. When
I was an unhappy and exceedingly lonely student at Yale, I
could identify almost everyone in my class of over one thousand
men because I had memorized our Class Directory from poring
over it so much, or from listening and observing so much from
the sidelines: This guy is from Shaker Heights and this one's
from La Jolla and that one went to Groton and that one grew
up in Switzerland and that one's father is a barber and that tall
guy's mother is a Du Pont. Few of them knew me. I didn't know

then that I would become a writer, and that this almost pathological interest in everybody's history would pursue me. Except
now it *is* pathological—"pertaining to or caused by disease."

Oh, how I, as a homosexual, have always loathed that word
"disease," and, worse, "caused by disease." I have fought so
hard—even to the point of not speaking to my sister-in-law,
Alice, for many months when, years ago, she said emphatically
that she knew homosexuality was an illness. "I just know it in
my heart of hearts," she said, looking me straight in the eye,
as I stood there speechless and fuming, having no ammunition
to fight back with, beyond the same argument: I knew, and
know, in *my* heart of hearts, that she's wrong. I was born just
as she was born.

And also—because AIDS has brought gay men much closer,
so that friendships that would ordinarily take years to develop
are now quickly made and cemented—those of us fighting this
epidemic find ourselves with many new friends very quickly
indeed. (It's not unusual to go to a funeral and find that most
of the mourners are men and women the deceased became
friendly with after his AIDS diagnosis.)

I believe most gay men now know more dead gay men than
they realize, or allow themselves to think about.

I only recently discovered that the number of dead I knew
was so great. For the first several years of this epidemic, I
dutifully kept a list in a little green notebook. When the number
reached two hundred, sometime in 1985, I stopped. I'm not quite
certain why. Even then it seemed hyperbolic to discuss such a
large number; or perhaps I was going through one of my periodic bouts of burnout, deciding enough was enough. But I
didn't really stop. When I came across an obituary anywhere of
someone I knew, I'd clip it out and toss it into a box. When I
heard another name in conversations, on the phone, walking
down the street, at dinners or other social gatherings, I'd make
a note of the name on a piece of paper and toss that into the box
too. (Listening to conversations of gay men at social gatherings
recently, I've realized how completely we've come to absorb the
morbidity of our lives; men pass along information of deaths
casually interspersed in the flow of whatever else they're talking about, as in "He's got a new Volvo, Peter must have left
him some money, he says it's the best car he's ever had," or

"Frank got the house when Terry died, and Frank and Tom, his lover died . . . was it in August . . . are going to Europe, I got them into the Connaught in August, you know how hard it is to get anyone into the Connaught in August. . . ." These quotes come from men still in their twenties and thirties.)

When I started to write this essay, I pulled out the box and dumped the pieces of paper on the floor. I transferred the names and taped the obituaries onto three-by-five file cards, and then copied all the names from the green notebook onto file cards, too. I began to be aware that the task was taking me longer than I thought it would. Then I alphabetized them all, as best I could, because a number of the dead men were identified not with names, which I couldn't remember, but with descriptive phrases: "Alice's hairdresser"; "the guy I had a date with after the opening night of *No, No, Nanette*"; "Bruce Kaye's lover"; "the brother of the *Newsweek* reporter, they both came here to talk"; "the short doctor with the Italian name who was a friend of DW's [a man I was desperately in love with in 1975]"; "Coconut Grove—the guy with the Spanish first name and the Jewish last name"; "the kid who became an Orthodox Jew when he got sick, and then got married." I can still see most of their faces, even though I'm no longer as good with names as I was at Yale. After completing this task, I began asking friends to list for me names they remembered, and when I recognized one I didn't have, I added it to my own list. It was only when I counted the cards after I'd done all of this that I was startled to discover I had about five hundred. Just as startling is the knowledge that there are always more to be added. I continue to hear new names of acquaintances and friends I hadn't included. And *The New York Times* comes out every day.

(I used to encourage friends who were dating to settle down into relationships. I wasn't a matchmaker—just a romantic egging-on from the sidelines, hoping others would find what I hadn't. While filing my index cards, it upset me to note several couples I'd encouraged who had perhaps then infected each other.)

The publication that the Centers for Disease Control, the government agency responsible for monitoring this epidemic, puts out with the latest numbers, the latest physical

manifestations and permutations—for there are many illnesses
and diseases all under the category AIDS—is called the *Morbidity and Mortality Weekly Report*. The *MMWR*. On last
(1988) June 5th (the date, in 1981, that the *MMWR* first listed
cases of what was eventually to be named AIDS and, by this
inclusion, officially designated it an "epidemic"), this country
entered the eighth year of the AIDS epidemic. There is no cure.
There is still marked uncertainty about what is going on inside
our bodies. There is, among some of us, a growing conviction
that what we're told *is* going on may perhaps not be accurate.
Despite congressional appropriations—at last—of hundreds of
millions of dollars that would seem to dispute this, there is still
monumental indifference on the part of the straight world to
addressing this catastrophe, and predictions for the future are
even more grotesque than the numbers I live with now.

Figures, which all Americans, myself evidently included,
wallow in, from TV ratings to increased sales of gourmet take-
out, aren't really meaningful to me any longer. The figure "five
hundred" seems unreal. Death as a profound philosophical subject is currently ridiculous. Even now, in its non-philosophical
form, it's impossible to grasp, to get hold of, this unreality, just
somehow to live with it. With an average of several deaths a
week (there is a new American case diagnosed every fourteen
minutes), how could anyone? There's no time for grief or
mourning, certainly not for contemplation. I can't cry easily
anymore anyway. Phone calls advising me of another departure
from this world are too routine. As is finding familiar names in
the obits of the *Times*. I read the latest overall tallies. They're
awful. Everything's awful. And it's been awful for so long.

Over a year ago, I set out to write something—I wasn't
quite certain what. I'd submitted a proposal to several publications. I wanted to write regularly about AIDS, stories that
weren't being written and that I felt demanded to be written.
The AIDS epidemic is enormously complicated. It's so complicated that few reporters appear to understand what's going on.
I consider all AIDS reporting everywhere, without exception,
to be imprecise and superficial. The latest news, be it a medical
or scientific discovery or a proposed legislative action—each
and all tied in knotted strands of potential controversy (usually
including either the word "discriminatory" or "mandatory")—

cannot be encapsulated in one-minute segments on the evening news or even in 1,400 words, which newspapers occasionally, at the limits of their generosity, allocate. And I think something very grim has happened to American journalism: It has become bland and increasingly conservative. The sort of deep, investigative reporting that I grew up with and took for granted has apparently disappeared. I was tired of calling my reporter contacts, pointing out the AIDS scandals they weren't writing about, and watching them still not write about them. Or reading their articles and calling them up to say they'd missed the point. Or writing them lengthy letters critiquing their articles in detail. Or berating them for not bothering to get a statement from someone representing another point of view. Most AIDS reporters seem to think there is only one point of view: that promulgated by the United States government and its many agencies dealing with the epidemic (but not with each other). I thought I'd better stop complaining about this and do it myself—that, as a writer and someone well acquainted with this awful drama and its huge cast of characters, I could be most effective in this way.

My proposal was accepted by a large newspaper and its syndicate. I went to Washington for a month, to research my first article. I decided I wanted to write about the total lack of any AIDS chain of command, the fact that nobody was really in charge, and the complete disarray among those who were meant to be involved—to try to make readers understand that, in these circumstances, little would get done. I wrote the article, which appeared in the "home" newspaper I was attached to by the syndicate, and then I became despondent as I silently watched it not picked up at all when it was wired—two times— in full to some 300 newspapers across the country, wired in summary to some 1,200 newspapers across the country, and even when the syndicate salesman personally made an appeal to his twelve leading newspapers.

But that is not the point of *this* essay, beyond demonstrating how hard it is for the gay community to get our story out to the straight world. All writers are familiar with rejection. The point that *is* applicable, that I do want to make, is that in my discouragement I quit. Instead of persevering and hoping that the forthcoming articles, as sometimes happens, would begin to accrue additional syndicated outlets, I absorbed my rejection and frustration and took my marbles and went home.

As with the mounting tallies of lost friends, those of us who have been trying to confront this losing battle seem to have an infinite capacity not only to absorb the worst, but to be defeated by it. So many deaths have not turned very many of us into fighters. We are all, naturally, infinitely tired ("AIDSed-out" is the expression). Whatever energy can be summoned to fight perceived wrongs has, for many, long since dribbled away.

That it's taken over a year for me to sit down and tackle this project again is less a token of my energy or commitment, or my ability to overcome my conviction that whatever I write will again fall on deaf ears, or my renewed energy after a period of burnout, than it is of my realizing again that there's nothing else to do. There's nothing else important enough to write about. I should be making a living writing something that might produce for me the income I need like everyone else (my brother, Arthur, only half-jokingly remarks that I'm using AIDS as an excuse *not* to work and write), but I don't have the interest or energy for that kind of writing. What actually gets me started again is not the inspiration (I am sorry to say that the loss of five hundred no longer works, as it once did, as the more-than-sufficient inspiration), but the realization that over a year has passed. Where did that year go? How many three-by-fives? (About ninety.) How many more of us became infected? What dynamite will ever ignite experimental drug-testing at the Food and Drug Administration and at the National Institutes of Health, of the more than two hundred promising treatments that "CBS Evening News" casually mentioned recently were available somewhere else in the world but not here? What did I do with my life for one whole year? Oh, I know what I did—but what did I *do?*

In other words, I became frightened again. If, as I fear, my days are probably numbered, how can I afford to be so wasteful of time? I was brought up a Jew, by two intelligent parents, both professionals (my father a lawyer and my mother a social worker), and fifty-three years of the instilled necessity to achieve does not disappear, especially, it would seem, in the face of death.

Why do I feel I have to offer these excuses? Excuses for

what? For my year of inactivity or for my decision, once again, to try to write about this? I haven't been completely honest with you. I did not waste a year doing nothing. I wrote two plays. I put together a book of my political writings of these AIDS years. I rewrote a screenplay of my play *The Normal Heart*, about the early years of the epidemic. That is certainly a good year's work, by any standards, Jewish or otherwise. Why do I discount it so?

Because none of it has any meaning for today, now, this minute? How can that be? I ache for *The Normal Heart* to be a film, because there have been no motion pictures, yet and still, documenting these years of horror. One of the new plays is a farce "inspired by" some of those I consider monstrously responsible for the AIDS predicament—the First Family and the Mayor of A Large City. The other play, a companion piece to *The Normal Heart*, which I call *The Furniture of Home*, is about growing up with my parents and my brother, covering some forty years; its theme, which evidently provided enough energetic fuel for me to write it, can be stated simply: You spend so many years fighting to come to terms with being homosexual, you finally not only accept yourself but like yourself, and then the fucking plague comes along.

All of this work contains ideas I want people to hear. So why do I disparage it? Do I feel guilty because I'm not fighting this fight twenty-four hours a day? Do I feel guilty I'm alive?

I come back to my opening sentence: I don't think any heterosexual can understand what it's like to be a homosexual man today. I somehow want every heterosexual to understand that. I want my brother and sister-in-law to understand that.

I am presently, as I write this sentence, in various stages of estrangement from both of them because of a recent example of my "gay activist" behavior. I wrote a strong and threatening letter to a large corporate client of Arthur's firm to protest their unjust firing of a gay employee; Arthur and Alice took great offense at my involving Arthur in this way. You must know that my brother has always been the most important person in my life and that our devotion to each other has been total; like the only two members of a fraternity, we have prided ourselves, in our adult lives, on our closeness, in the eyes of the world as well as our own. We would have lunch regularly once a week; then—

with the arrival of AIDS and my increasing political activism—
this became less regular, supplanted by weekly phone calls
back and forth. Both calls and lunches have now become spo-
radic and suffused with forced casualness. Before I wrote the
letter, I had asked him for advice on how to write it. Homosexuality is the only subject between us that, even after some thirty-
five years of knowing about mine, he cannot talk about
comfortably. An edge of upset comes into his voice, which rises
a pitch or two, an edge that I recognize as not only discomfort
but anger—that I've brought the subject up or that he doesn't
want to talk about it, I don't know which. Probably both. And
the rejection that I instantly feel evokes my own hardly sup-
pressed anger: Even after some thirty-five years of knowing
this does that to him, I slam down the phone. And wait for him
to call back. Which he always has done, so far. It is exceedingly
painful for me to confront the possibility that my very own
brother might have to be included in that "straight" world for
which I find myself having less and less tolerance.

Recently, before this episode, in the course of chatting
about many things, including AIDS—for I make a determined
effort to force the subject down his and Alice's and our mother's
throats—he casually asked me, "You're worried about your
health?"

That he could have asked me such a question, eight years
into an epidemic that has taken many of my friends whom he
knew, and despite his cognizance of my political involvement,
and my writings which I've seen to it he's had copies of, and the
organizations I helped to start, to one of which I finagled him
into becoming pro bono legal adviser, and the massive media
coverage (even if I don't think they're the right stories, at last
now there are plenty of stories) has, as our mother puts it when
she stews about something that upsets her, "stuck in my craw."

What does he think I worry about? To watch friend after
friend be taken from me to die after ghastly and punishing
illnesses and not be frightened? To see dread spots erupt over-
night on previously unblemished skins and limbs of still-living
other friends and not be frightened? To hear incipient coughs
transmute from hacking barks into sudden silence and not be
frightened? I guess this sounds melodramatic. And my prose

has turned purple too. Am I begging for sympathy? Yes. Am I begging for help? Yes. Am I frightened? You bet your life.

In the end, I realize I can't write about anything else. Every story is the same story. What I have written this past year is the only thing I can write now. Primo Levi, the survivor of Auschwitz who somehow managed to write magnificently of his horrible memories, said in *If This Is a Man* (reprinted as *Survival in Auschwitz*): "The need to tell our story to 'the rest,' to make 'the rest' participate in it, had taken on for us . . . the character of an immediate violent impulse, to the point of competing with other elementary needs."

Several months ago I met the first man I have allowed myself to make love with, and be (safely) intimate with, and consider having a relationship with—in five years. Luke. I have not made love in five years. One of the last men I loved died from AIDS in 1983. Men who have been romantically important in my life in earlier, pre-AIDS years (there's no margin of safety in thinking like this: the putative causal virus might have an incubation period of twenty years) have also died. It is very difficult for me to make love, even "safely," when the very act is now so inextricably bound up with death. I don't mean the memory of my dead lover, though that, too, of course, is there. (I have undergone periodic satisfactory tests on my body's immune system—though not for HIV, because I consider this test, perhaps irrationally, unconvincing. It's not that I disbelieve its probable efficacy, it's just that I still don't believe *enough* to subject myself to living under such a sword of Damocles. To be fair, I must say that I have many friends whose opinions I respect who consider my refusal to be tested for HIV a state of denial.) I mean the very act itself—of kissing, of gently masturbating each other, of sweating bodies lying side by side. All the educational material in the world proclaiming that "safe sex" is possible does not reduce the fear that some slipup might occur. Is it fatal if his semen on my hand enters the tiny exposed cuticle under a minuscule hangnail on my thumb? Or my sweat into his scraped knee (he belongs to a gay wrestling team)? Is kissing really safe? I know they say it is, that no cases have been discovered that result from kissing, but do they really know? How do you define "kissing"?

How do you draw distinctions between kisses and kisses? There are reported cases of single-contact infection. Contact with what, exactly, and where? Anal intercourse is considered to be the most dangerous activity. But I know dead men who never engaged in it. So many hard-and-fast dicta have been issued at some time during these years of scientific and epidemiological investigation, only to be refuted, contradicted, contravened days, weeks, months, or years later. And so many of the men and women making these pronouncements I know to be, from personal encounters, truly second-rate (many first-rate minds have refused to participate), or corseted by ironclad requirements of a bureaucracy determined, at any cost, not to create panic in "the general population." (Before 1981, I'd always considered myself a part of "the general population." But before 1981, I also believed in democracy.) So it's difficult for me to believe anything.

And yet I found myself falling in love. Like other human beings, I desire the experience. I wanted to hold this man and to kiss him. Is this wanting too much? Is this wanting too much *now?* Can any straight person understand what it is like to want to make love but to be terrified that to do so means possible death? Even breaking the most stringent and necessary diet for one's health doesn't kill you; you have a binge and go back on the diet tomorrow, plagued only with guilt. It took me many years of psychoanalysis to rid myself of guilts—over being homosexual, over not being as financially successful as my brother, over . . . oh, the endless agenda of what we think the world expects of us that we're not fulfilling; now guilt creeps back in yet another door. I feel guilty falling in love. I should have more control over my emotions. I don't want to die. I have important work to try to do quickly, before I die. I don't want to die.

I want to live and I want to love and I want, in the universal as well as the specific sense, all my brothers to try to understand why this epidemic is here—because I think there are reasons why it is here—and, with your understanding, to help us, for we, and I, desperately need help. That's why I'm writing this. For Arthur and Alice and for every heterosexual friend I find myself hating, when I don't want to hate.

And in so writing, perhaps I can also try to offer thoughts on some questions:

■ Why are homosexuals not allowed to state that many of us *know* we are born homosexual, as straight men are born heterosexual, as bisexual men are born bisexual, without such staunch opposition from so many others, on so many fronts? Why is it so important to *them* that this cannot be so? What is their vested interest in keeping us sick? And illegal?

■ Why has the straight world, by and large, been unable to face or cope with the realities of what is happening to us—to such a degree that I now believe some form of intentional genocide is going on?

■ Why have not more gay men fought against the world's intolerance of us, the way we are treated, in just about every way? Why do gay men accept the decisions of others so passively?

■ Are gay men, cooperating with the System, being the "good little boys" we were brought up to be, helping to kill our own? Are organizations like GMHC *in any way* like the Jewish councils set up during World War II to help the Germans exterminate them?

II

In May 1987, prior to my trip to Washington to research my article, I made these notes, using information published in *The New Internationalist,* a British magazine published in Oxford:

The World Health Organization estimates that some 50,000 people around the world have so far died as a result of AIDS, with a further 50,000 terminally ill. To many experts, this figure of 100,000 cases in all is a conservative figure. What we do know, from statistics compiled over five years in many different countries, is that for every full-blown case of AIDS there are *at least* one hundred carriers of the infection who have not as yet developed the disease. Of these one hundred, at least ten already have come down with ARC—AIDS-Related Complex. If we accept the World Health Organization's figure of 100,000 AIDS cases, then this implies that there are a million people in the world with ARC, and 10 million carrying the putative virus. The World Health Organization's 100,000 dead or dying from AIDS today becomes 10 million dead or dying by the year 2000.

And, again, WHO's figure is conservative. Research in Africa strongly suggests that 10 percent of the 100-million population of the worst-affected central zone are now carriers of the putative virus: In other words, there are, at this minute, 10 million infected *in Central Africa alone.* Add to this the infection in the rest of the world, including the United States, with an estimated 2.6 million carriers—also thought to be a very conservative estimate (Dr. Robert Gallo, of the National Cancer Institute, claimed, in the London *Observer* in April *1985,* that two million were already infected)—and we obtain, according to WHO, a current global figure of 15 million or more people infected with the putative virus. All these people are infectious as well as infected, capable of passing on a virus to others with whom they have sexual contact. So 15 million infected today implies a great many more infected a year from now and the year after that. Indeed, the World Health Organization estimates a world total of *100 million* infected within five to ten years.

One year later, at the Fourth International AIDS Conference in Stockholm, these figures have been more than generously confirmed.

I won't dwell on the possibility that troubles me and a few others: that HIV is not the *only* cause of AIDS, that it's possible it isn't, that there's a cofactor, or an additional cause, or additional causes, or that HIV might be only a marker (and a marker not 100-percent present), or not the cause at all. Though many scientists everywhere claim HIV is the only cause, there are a few distinguished ones who now maintain otherwise.

And I won't dwell on this either: That, for reasons I find incomprehensible, the non-African world and the straight white population in America and elsewhere seem to put enormous confidence in an unproved theory: that AIDS cannot happen to them. That something "different" is going on in Africa and gay (and now parts of black and Hispanic) America. That viruses discriminate. (Heterosexual Americans, both white and black, prefer to ignore what's happening in Africa, setting up yet another prejudice.)

And they ignore a proved theory: that this putative virus appears to have an incubating latency of, so far as is known at present, up to twenty years. If this is so, it would not be inconceivable that someone with whom one had sex twenty years ago might have passed along the virus.

Why doesn't it make sense to them that what's happening now in Central Africa began much earlier in time? Why doesn't it make sense to them that gay men's AIDS and drug-related AIDS are just another stage, as Central Africa is an earlier one?

For every "expert" public official who has proclaimed that "the general population" need not be concerned, there's a medical or epidemiological or scientific "expert" (who, more often than not, is not interviewed or on television) who just as emphatically proclaims that a virus has no way of knowing who's black or white or straight or gay.

I don't want this essay to be a compilation of damning statistical predictions. Surely we've learned by now that just about any argument, no matter how extreme, can be supported by "statistics." (I consider most epidemiologists to be, along with insider traders, major gonifs.) At the worst, even providing mountains of horrible evidence, as Jonathan Kozol recently did in preparing his moving and cogent exposé of the homeless in New York City, appears to result in nothing beyond a blizzard of numbers and facts and details falling on an uncaring world. The ability of exposés to ignite action seems to have diminished substantially in recent years. It's almost as if we have not only seen the worst, but we now expect it. It (whatever "it" stands for) is not going to change. There's been a little spurt of a reaction of disgust recently to this Age of Greed we live in, particularly in New York, where the two extremes are extraordinarily noticeable; but it seems only a spurt, and a long way from being revolutionary enough to turn the landowners off their land. The downtrodden are weak, not angry. There doesn't seem to be very much anger around these days, but there is a lot of exhaustion or, worse, acceptance. I watch too many PBS documentaries about those who "fall through the cracks." These documentaries all seem to wind up with someone saying something like, "The future will judge what kind of people we were by how we took care of_____." Fill in the blank with your own favorite set of problems.

In a letter defending herself against an attack "on my political views and my personal motives," the philosopher Hannah Arendt responded: "What Mr. Halpern, like many of our politically interested intellectuals, does not understand is that we deal in politics with warnings and not with prophecies. If I were foolish and resigned enough to play the role of prophet, I certainly should also be content to share his eternal fate, which is to be proved wrong time and again, except at the decisive moment, when it is too late."

The figures I have cited are not prophecies of doom, "only" warnings. Why do people refuse to hear warnings?

Why is it that white heterosexuals prefer not to think about or deal with AIDS? For the African and the black and Hispanic American cases, it's because of racism. For the gay male cases, it's because of homophobia.

III

I wonder why so many gays demand that our lives and experiences be viewed "positively," when in fact we have lived through such horrors to get here. Jews demand, of themselves and the world, constant remembrance of their tortured history. Homosexuals have been hated by religion, state, country, world, and history, by parents and families and peers. (This is a horrible singularity of the gay situation: Can Jews imagine being hated *by their parents* for their Jewishness?) If a writer, gay or straight, attempts to detail the fallout from these experiences in his work, accusations of "self-hate," "negativism," or the worst offense, of course, "homophobia"—which, when leveled by one gay against another, brings the charge full circle back to "self-hate"—are the automatic, knee-jerk responses. Why are we so insistent on wringing only joy and laughter out of our painful history—to such an extreme degree that we now pride ourselves in naming ourselves and what we are "gay"?

Perhaps because I am both, I find it remarkable how many similarities I notice between homosexuals and Jews. I turn for support for these convictions of mine to Hannah Arendt. History recently made a pretty good attempt to destroy the Jewish people, and as I think history now has an opportunity to do (and is already doing) pretty much the same to homosexuals, there are obvious lessons to be learned in a study of her work.

It would be interesting to know what Hannah Arendt (who died in 1975) thought of the Italian chemist and writer, Primo Levi. "Anyone who has been tortured remains tortured," Levi quotes a friend tortured by the Gestapo who committed suicide some thirty years later. Levi, in his last book, *The Drowned and the Saved*, published in 1986, before his own apparent suicide in 1987, attempts to establish hierarchies of innocence and guilt among both the victims and the victimizers. Levi concluded it was possible to be "less guilty." I doubt Arendt would allow this.

It is fascinating how harsh Arendt is in her etiology of modern anti-Semitism. She looks no further than her own front door. As the Princeton professor George Kateb writes in his book, *Hannah Arendt—Politics, Conscience, Evil:* "She argues that antisemitism could not have become the elemental force that it became . . . unless the Jews themselves had something to do with it."

She asks, as I ask of gay people: Why are we so hated? Why are we disliked? Why do we make so many uncomfortable? Why do we particularly offend the "good family man" Arendt describes so disparagingly as the great modern criminal, who would do anything to save his family, up to and including murder (Adolf Eichmann)?

In our case, I can understand some of the reasons for the repugnance felt by the "good family man": to start with, we gays are perceived to have what he doesn't and fantasizes he desires—freedom, sexual choice without commitment, continued unlimited sexual choice (until eight years ago). We are perceived to be utterly and totally promiscuous, even though for most of us this description has always been far from accurate. But again, particularly during and after the "swinging sixties" (and seventies), into which the heterosexual populations were also released with abandon, this stereotype took hold, in full disregard of that overwhelming majority of us who were either in monogamous relationships or just as inept or frightened of sex as everyone else. But it seemed to serve the straight world's purpose, and perhaps our own, to be seen as so sexually athletic. It's certainly more manly than being seen as a sissy.

For reasons as incomprehensible to me as the ancient "reasons" for hating Jews (that they drank the blood of Christian children), I don't understand the irrational fear that apparently grips so many parents of school-age children, that we will "recruit" these children. (And why is there never fear that straight male teachers will seduce little girls?) Study after study has proved that gays are not child molesters, that child molesters are overwhelmingly heterosexual, and yet the belief persists. (Although curiously no one goes after the Catholic Church, where so much of the priesthood *is* gay; I have few Catholic friends who weren't aware of this when they were young. As Dr. Robert J. Stoller remarks in his generally inadequate entry on homosexuality in the *Encyclopaedia Britannica:* "To the church's discomfort, those most able to abstain from heterosexuality may lean toward homosexuality.") I know of no gay people who enjoy seeking sexual relations with someone who is not gay; it simply isn't a gay characteristic. So this myth of recruitment, like the belief that all gay men are promiscuous, must serve some purpose for the straight world—to keep us different and dangerous—and the dangerous must always be watched and rallied against, to the extent of law.

(In those instances where children do have sex with their homosexual elders, be they teachers or anyone else, I submit that often, very often, the child desires the activity, and perhaps even solicits it, either because of a natural curiosity that will or will not develop along these lines, or because he or she is homosexual and innately knows it. This is far from "recruitment." Obviously, there are instances in which the child is unwilling, and is a victim of sexual abuse, homo- or heterosexual. But, as with straight children anxious for the experience with someone of the opposite sex, there are kids who seek, solicit, and consent willingly to sex with someone of the same sex. And, unlike girls or women forced into rape and traumatized, most gay men have warm memories of their earliest and early sexual encounters; when we share these stories with each other, they are invariably positive ones. What has not been positive is our knowledge, from that early date, of the world's disapproval. I realize that this is a very volatile issue, and that this in no way absolves the adult participant of responsibility in colluding in such acts, be it with boys or girls. Nor am I sanctioning sex with children, most of which I personally find as abhorrent as if I was a parent of a child myself. I am just saying that the issue is not so cut-and-dried as many laws and many parents and many righteous moralists maintain.)

As with all kinds of sex, attempts at prevention aren't going to stop them. They only increase the quotient of guilt and self-loathing—results exceptionally costly, both in economic terms and those of mental health. Most gay people knew they were gay from a very early age, whether they acted on it or not. Not only have we always known it, but we also know what many don't wish to hear: that we can't change and, more important, most of us don't want to change—just as heterosexuals can't change and, more important, don't want to change. Why can't society accept what we've known for so long, that sexuality is a *given?* I know I am stating a blasphemous heresy to too many when I say this. I'll be coming back to it later.

Many gay kids are now discovering their homosexuality earlier, accepting it earlier, acting on it earlier, and, mercifully, becoming more comfortable with it earlier. It's now possible for gay kids to know other gay kids (something I never experienced) or, if not actually to know them, at least to see them portrayed on television or read about them in newspapers or novels. It's no longer necessary to think you're the only person in the world with these feelings. Of course, not all of these experiences are going to be positive; there is always going to be peer rejection, for instance. Yet, gradually, there are places for the young to go: youth organizations in cities like New York, and gay high school and college groups. The recent brouhaha that erupted among Yale alumni when an article in *The Wall Street Journal* correctly identified that university as having a large gay student population no doubt will be repeated in a growing number of other centers of higher learning. The still-continuing legal battle between the administration of Georgetown University and the city of Washington, D.C. (which has an antidiscrimination ordinance that protects homosexuals), over whether a gay student organization should be allowed on campus and funded like other student groups, will also no doubt be repeated elsewhere. What is also going to continue is the growing visibility of this young gay population. It becomes increasingly evident that many of them are not going to hide in the closet for most of their lives, as so many of their predecessors have done.

The concept of "manliness" is the stereotypical straight expectation for all males; somehow, all gay men are therefore "sissies." (How gay men hate this word!) As with all stereotypes, there are many examples to prove them true. But there are larger numbers that do not. (In a 1957 study, Dr. Evelyn Hooker demonstrated that less than 10 percent of gay men fulfill any stereotypical category.) Many effeminate men are totally heterosexual, and many gay men are indistinguishable from their straight brothers. But it is the stereotypes which are seen, photographed, televised. When Gay Pride parades are photographed across the country in late June, it's always the few gays in outlandish costumes who catch the eye of the media. The hundreds of thousands who look just like everybody's son or daughter or husband or wife are not so visually titillating.

If all gay men are sissies, the stereotypical reasoning follows, then all gay men wear dresses. This makes little sense. As Brian McNaught, a gay counselor and teacher, points out, why would a *man* who is attracted to *men* and wants to be attractive to *men* wear a dress?

Over the last fifteen years, gay men have worked very hard to change their perceived image. The 1970s were years of "clonedom." Levi 501 jeans (the kind with the button flies), work boots, flannel shirts, mustaches, beards, and bodies heavily muscled from constant gymnasium workouts were all requirements for this look; we *were* the Marlboro men. (Indeed we were the model, the prototype, for the Marlboro man— straight men across the country were soon copying *us,* and now television and movies are filled with the mustached, work-

booted, flannel-shirted, muscled "straight" man we made popular. As with the discos and disco music of this era that we also
popularized, the gay contribution to popular culture is an area
that sociologists have conveniently overlooked.) But, ironically,
this new look came to be just as stereotypical as the former
swish, limp-wristed model we were so anxious to replace—and
the very sight of a group of men wearing work boots, 501's, and
mustaches became just as gay-identifying, and just as likely to
produce the homophobic response of "look at those faggots."
(The standard shot used ad nauseum on television and in photo-
journalism, when homosexuality or anything about the gay
community is discussed, is that of two men, shot from behind,
with their arms around each other, their hands on each other's
Levied asses.)

Non-Jews also embrace stereotypes when hating Jews:
Jews are moneylenders; Jews are criminals; Jews are greedy;
Jews are more loyal to each other than to the outside world;
Jews, through secret cabals, control the world. All Jews are
dark and hirsute. All Jews are Shylock or Fagin. All Jews are
smarter, more ambitious. All of these stereotypes could be perceived as being somehow interconnected, pollen from the same
plant. They all involve money, greed, power. Even that favorite
Christian slander hurled at Jews—that they killed Christ—can
be conceived as an attempt to maintain power.

On the surface, gay stereotypes don't seem to blend so well.
For instance, at the same time that we are perceived as amusing, decorative, effeminate, and creative (I often think that the
entire gay population is considered to be composed of nothing
but hairdressers and interior decorators), we are perceived as
being sexually threatening to children, or to husbands and
wives. It doesn't seem to occur to many that foppishness and
sexual prowess are an unlikely combination. And our sexual
"threats" seem to provoke peculiar, contrary reactions: I've
heard of wives who are far more upset when they lose their
husbands to another man than to another woman, when she
should be less so—it has little to do with her, or what she might
have been or done. But, instead, she often sees this rejection as
some sort of challenge: She will "change" him. Indeed, I know
straight women who pursue gay men for just this reason (when
in actuality this pursuit might reflect the woman's desire not to

have a sexual relationship at all). Too, the woman who enjoys
the company of the amusing gay man because he is amusing is
usually less interested in the straight man because he isn't. (It
was Proust who pointed out that the homosexual was one of the
few members of society not bored to death and still capable of
passions.) The pool of available, eligible, interesting and interested straight men, for some women, is often limited, and they
turn to gay male friends for companionship; such women, unkindly termed "fag hags," are seen quite often in large cities
like New York. So gay men would seem to serve as less of a
threat than a convenience.

Here is a short compilation of responses I've received when
I've asked people, both gay and straight, why they think homosexuals are hated. Invariably the first thought is that people
hate *difference.* Anything that veers from the norm. Anything
that veers from the rigid family way. (It seems slightly ludicrous that gays not procreating should be considered—in this
age of woeful overpopulation—as a reason for disapproval.) An
inability to perceive differences: They're frightened because
they *can't* see us, they can only sense our threat. People aren't
flexible in general. (Look at how many churches have bounda-
ries on what is acceptable sex.) They don't see multiple points
of view as being an option. They see black and white without
many shades of gray in between. We're hitting people where
they live their most secret terrors. My niece, Liza, a graduate
student in English literature, said, "It's just too threatening:
People can't deal with that part of themselves, because I think
everybody has homosexual as well as heterosexual feelings."
Straights are shackled to their families and family values,
which we flagrantly disavow. It's not unlike racism and anti-
Semitism or sexism. (Gay women are not nearly so ostracized
as gay men. Here is a bit of perverse sexism: women's sexuality
is considered unimportant, therefore not a threat.) We go
against the theory of capitalism (say some on the gay left): We
produce no children to become workers. (But capitalism breaks
up the family, sending women and children away from their
homes.) Everyone has a *need* for a scapegoat—a way of not
facing their own problems and responsibilities. The heterosexual majority must be in control; they're going to oppress all
who, in any way, threaten their power (their beliefs).

While each of these reasons could no doubt serve as the basis for an entire book, I think they don't get to the root cause, but are rather manifestations, perhaps even rationalizations, of it.

Hannah Arendt believed quite simply, as Professor Kateb puts it, that "modern antisemitism depends on the character of modern Jews." Arendt talks about the two main Jewish responses to anti-Semitism, the parvenu and the pariah. The parvenu tried to become assimilated at all costs, and the pariah was an outcast, who accepted his position as an outcast. Either way aggravated anti-Semitism.

Arendt begins *Antisemitism,* the first part of her monumental trilogy *The Origins of Totalitarianism,* with a thought so simple as to be shocking. Who has ever thought of this?: "There is hardly an aspect of contemporary history more irritating and mystifying than the fact that of all the great unsolved political questions of our century, it should have been this seemingly small and unimportant Jewish problem that had the dubious honor of setting the whole infernal machine in motion." The "infernal machine" obviously is World War II. By then European Jews had long since lost what power they had accumulated, despite the Nazis' claim that it was Jewish world political power that must serve as the pretext for killing them off. Arendt goes all the way back to "Tocqueville's great discovery" that "wealth without visible function is much more intolerable because nobody can understand why it should be tolerated." Translated to the situation prior to World War II, this meant: "Antisemitism reached its climax when Jews had similarly lost their public functions and their influence, and were left with nothing but their wealth."

Arendt makes a clear distinction between anti-Semitism and Jew-hating, which always existed but, in those years of Jewish power, only on an unofficial, behind-the-back basis. When Jews lost this power, it was all right for Jew-hating to be officially codified as anti-Semitism. So long as any group has power, it's not in the majority's interest to crucify or cremate its members. But "wealth without power or aloofness without a policy are felt to be parasitical, useless, revolting, because such conditions cut all the threads which tie men together."

For a moment, Arendt turns aside: "Just as antisemites

understandably desire to escape responsibility for their deeds, so Jews, attacked and on the defensive, even more understandably do not wish under any circumstances to discuss their share of responsibility." Why are Jews responsible? Because they "avoided all political action for two thousand years." They are a people without a government, without a country, without one language. Despite the elements of their faith, which did contain well-defined concepts of history and moral philosophy, they spent two thousand years avoiding anything remotely resembling political action to defend and protect themselves or their beliefs. "The result was that the political history of the Jewish people became even more dependent upon unforeseen, accidental factors than the history of other nations, so that the Jews stumbled from one role to the other and accepted responsibility for none." Since they never fought back, it became increasingly easy to punish, torture, and scapegoat them.

I think it can quite easily be maintained that gay people have been marching around the earth for just as long. We have not been united in the same way as Jews, although, as John Boswell, Professor of History at Yale, writes so cogently in his *Christianity, Social Tolerance, and Homosexuality*, once upon a time homosexuals were a distinct group, before the centuries of going underground. "Few classicists," Boswell writes, "have doubted that homosexuality occupied a prominent and respected position in most Greek and Roman cities at all levels of society and among a substantial portion of the population." Indeed, in ancient Greece, "many . . . writers use homosexual love as an ideal to which heterosexual lovers might aspire." In ancient Rome, "if Gibbon was right, the Roman Empire was ruled for almost two hundred consecutive years by men whose homosexual interests, if not exclusive, were sufficiently noteworthy to be recorded for posterity."

Concerning the "cause" of homosexuality, Professor Boswell has this to say: "There are in fact no explanations in any classical literature for homosexual desire, which everyone apparently considered ubiquitous and entirely ordinary." And this: "It should be noted that what 'causes' homosexuality is an issue of importance only to societies which regard gay people as bizarre or anomalous. Most people do not wonder what 'causes' statistically ordinary characteristics, like heterosexual desire or right-handedness; 'causes' are sought only for personal attributes which are assumed to be outside the ordinary pattern of life. Since very few in the ancient world considered homosexual behavior odd or abnormal, comments about its etiology were quite rare."

Boswell is also interested in comparing Jews and gays. "The fate of Jews and gay people has been almost identical throughout European history, from early Christian hostility to extermination in concentration camps. The same laws which oppressed Jews oppressed gay people; the same groups bent on eliminating Jews tried to wipe out homosexuality; the same periods of European history which could not make room for Jewish distinctiveness reacted violently against sexual nonconformity; the same countries which insisted on religious uniformity imposed majority standards of sexual conduct; and even the same methods of propaganda were used against Jews and gay people—picturing them as animals bent on the destruction of the children of the majority."

Boswell also mentions what he considers significant differences: Judaism is passed on consciously from parents to children, while gay people "suffer oppression individually and alone, without benefit of advice or frequently even emotional support from relatives or friends."

It is this same aloneness that many psychiatrists insist on using for their paradigm in not only repressing comparisons between the development of Jews and gay people, but also in denying gays anything approaching mental health and social equality. Therapists seem to compile identical lists: Gays did not have families to support them through the years of terror; we had no role models; we were rejected by our parents—in the case of gay men particularly by our fathers; we had so many early rejections from all and sundry as to think ourselves "dirty" and, indeed, morally wrong; therefore we have difficulty forming satisfactory relations with either one another or society; therefore we are ashamed of our homosexuality and hide it.

I submit that it's too easy to use this catalogue of possible truths to flog the mental health of homosexuals. There are Jewish families that are ashamed of being Jewish, that do not support each other against the world's intolerance of their differences, and instead try in every way to be accepted by those in majority. This is Arendt's own point, when she views parvenus with such antagonism: They, too, are denying who they are with misguided determination. Does this send them all to analytic couches? Did this make them sick in the eyes of psychiatry?

No, whatever else they were called, Jews were never thought of as "sick" by the majority, nor Judaism an illness. Where did this notion of homosexuality as an "illness" come from, and why has it persisted for so long? Boswell traces many centuries of "reasons." Most of them emanated from established religions, or from the seats of ruling power (which could, of course, be one and the same) and most of them had to do, not with the fear of "difference" cited by those I questioned, but with a determination on the part of an established interest to cement absolute power. But I am less interested in those early tyrants than in modern ones.

Freud himself considered homosexuality more an inconvenience than anything else. In an often-quoted letter to a worried mother, he said it would be easier, the world being the way it is, if one did not have to be homosexual. (One of these days, somebody ought to research fully Freud's own exceptionally close attachment to Wilhelm Fliess. It was certainly much more than just a friendship, and perhaps, noting this in himself, Freud passed on to other subjects for his scrutiny.) Dr. Stoller, in his *Encyclopaedia Britannica* article, (my edition is that of 1975), refers to "Freud's statement that all human beings possess undercurrents of homosexuality because they are biologically and thus psychologically bisexual." Why, then, did modern psychoanalysis take it upon itself to metamorphose "inconvenience"—indeed, "bisexual" tendencies—into illness? When did "the medicalization of homosexuality" take such a strong hold? The term "homosexual" appears to date from the late nineteenth century; the supplement (not published until 1976) to the unabridged *Oxford English Dictionary* (the main *OED*, published in 1933, does not include it) cites its first appearance as in *Psychopathia Sexualis* by Dr. Richard von Krafft-Ebing, a German neuropsychiatrist and early student of sexual psychopathology. That "ground-breaking examination of sexual aberrations" *(Encyclopaedia Britannica)*—in which just about everything except heterosexual intercourse in the missionary position is made to sound sufficient to ensure incarceration in the local nuthouse—was published in 1886.

It is my opinion that matters took a distinct turn for the worse with the arrival on these shores, from about 1930 on, of Freud's "children," mostly German analysts and mostly Jewish, in need of scapegoats of their own, and finding no others (particularly no others in numbers able to afford their services), they slowly institutionalized us homosexuals, in one way if not another. These German doctors were refugees themselves, and their own insecurities forged a great need to prove to the New World that they would fit in completely. It is perversely interesting to record that, of all the branches of modern therapy, most of which have come to accept the existence of so many gay people as sufficient evidence that nothing sick or abnormal is going on, the entrenched Freudians, in their network of Psychoanalytic Institutes located in each major American geographical area, are still the aggressive purveyors of this homosexuality-as-illness theme. (Boswell, in an unpublished paper, makes a very convincing comparison between today's psychiatrists and yesterday's priests; both have looked upon themselves as the only authorized keepers of the world's "morality.") How truly perverse: The persecuted now turned into persecutors.

That we gays don't pass on our "religion" from generation to generation is also, like aloneness, not a sufficient reason for preventing comparison with Jews. It is more than balanced by the fact that—no matter what methods are utilized to deny or expunge us—10 percent of any and every population will fall into Kinsey's homosexual category. So we are, in essence, self-perpetuating in a way even more reliable than the Jews' religious instruction of their young, which is not always so automatically self-perpetuating as Jewish elders like to think.

Most psychiatric literature, it seems to me, is written by men and women based only on their observations of those who come for treatment. There are many heterosexuals who had poor role models, were rejected by one or both parents, were rejected by many, all, or sundry, and who thought themselves "dirty" for one reason or another. Some become neurotic; many don't. The continued insistence by those who should now know better, like my brother and sister-in-law (for at last the psychiatric literature now has a growing number of works to refute it), that homosexuality is "caused" by an over-possessive mother and a rejecting or absent father, is no longer tolerable. Some 24 million gay men and women cannot all be here because of bad parenting: The number is simply too huge. I know too many gay men who loved their fathers and were loved by them in return. Or who had no mothers. Or who rejected the mothers they had. I know too many gay men and women who had and continue to have warm and loving families. I know plenty who haven't, but I know plenty of heterosexuals who haven't either. Homosexuality is not, in and of itself, the problem that causes gay people to seek treatment. It is the world's response to homosexuality. That and that alone is the "trouble" with homosexuality.

This response continues to be inhumanly perplexing in the light of so many scientific studies by notable academics, studies that have been generally accepted as valid. Dr. Alfred Kinsey, in 1948, startled the world with figures that have yet to be attacked or disproved. He said that 10 percent of American men were pretty much homosexual, that 4 percent of American men were exclusively homosexual, that 37 percent of American men had had a homosexual experience leading to orgasm post-puberty, and that 50 percent of American men have homosexual fantasies. Studies by Clellan S. Ford and Frank A. Beach, an anthropologist and a psychologist, found, in 1951, that homosexuality was accepted as normal in 64 percent of primitive societies, and in 1957, that homosexuality exists in every species of every mammal and that as the cortex of the brain develops, i.e., as creatures get smarter, the percentage of homosexuals increases. (This latter study is cited by Brian McNaught in *On Being Gay.*)

Surely it makes sense that if all mammals can be homosexual so naturally, these acts must be innate rather than learned. At least it does to me. Why is heterosexuality considered innate, an existential given, and not homosexuality? Or, if homosexuality is *learned*, why isn't heterosexuality *learned?* Homosexuality's attackers can't have their cake and eat it too. Even some gay people are unwilling to concede that they were born gay. One friend of mine says, "Your sexuality is deter-

mined by your third year." But another friend rebuts: "I know
some three-year-olds who sure know how to dress."

Homosexuals are born, just as heterosexuals are born. This
is what I think, feel, know, and there has been no evidence to
prove otherwise.

I offer this rephrasing of Arendt's notion: There is hardly an
aspect of contemporary history more irritating and mystifying
than the fact that of all the great unsolved political questions
of our century, it should have been this seemingly small and
unimportant problem of homosexuality that had the dubious
honor of setting the whole infernal machine in motion. Only this
time the "infernal machine" is the AIDS holocaust.

People hate victims, because they see in them something
they're terrified of becoming: themselves as victims. People
hate others for not doing what they themselves also feel powerless to do. All of this is embedded in the nineteenth-century
origins of anti-Semitism. European society and Western Jewry
disintegrated and declined pretty much together; there was no
balance of power between nations; there was no cooperation
between countries; and "the non-national, inter-European Jewish element became an object of universal hatred because of its
useless wealth, and of contempt because of its lack of power,"
both of which were now "atomized into a herd of wealthy individuals." Powerless non-Jews came to look upon wealthy
Jews not exercising the power commensurate with their wealth
as parasites.

I think that many heterosexuals look upon today's homosexuals in much the same way. Compared to most people, we appear to have large disposable incomes, we appear to exercise
few family or community responsibilities, we appear to be entirely frivolous and, until recently, utterly hedonistic, and this
hedonism has resulted in AIDS, which we are now expecting
the straight world to take care of immediately. Is it any wonder
that there is little sympathy for gay people and their plight?
This is Arendt's very point about the Jewish situation prior to
World War II.

For gays, this might appear in many ways a double-edged
sword, a situation of damned if you do, damned if you don't. We
hide because we know "they" don't like us; by our hiding,
"they" hate us even more. And the more we try to emerge from

our cocoon and into full view, the stronger are the forces prepared to slap us down and into hiding again. (I think it no
coincidence that the Jesse Helms amendment, refusing AIDS
funding to any organization that "advocated" or "promoted"
homosexuality, came immediately following the October 1987
March on Washington of some 650,000 gay men and lesbians.)
It's at this crucial juncture that we must realize that only by
capitalizing, in the many meanings of this word, on our coming
forth, can we save ourselves: When we capitalize on the power
inherent in our numbers, when we demand recognition in return for this power, only then will we not be murdered.

One of the richest men in America is gay; he is president of
one of the largest and wealthiest financial institutions in the
world; he is not known to be gay and shudders at the thought
that he'll be identified and revealed. This situation is repeated
across the country; in corporations, in banks, in businesses, in
family fortunes. If these gay men could unite, surely their
voices would be heard and answered in the corridors of power.

It is now a truism that every gay man who stays in the closet
is helping to kill the rest of his fellow gay men. Yet, instead of
provoking anger and hatred on the part of those who are "out"
against those still hiding within, it has fostered protection. We
all have our oppression in common and, like Vietnam veterans,
we've all been through various versions of the same war. We'll
take care of each other—even if, now, we are taking care of
those who help kill us. Their secret is safe with us.

I know there is historical reason for this—that the rite of
coming out is a precious and individual one, and that, in memory
of the pain it often entailed for so many, we honor each person's
privacy. But for a growing number of gay people, the maintenance of this protection is becoming increasingly more difficult
to sanction, either philosophically or pragmatically.

I offer as an example the late Terry Dolan, founder of the
National Conservative Political Action Committee, a PAC devoted exclusively to raising money for the conservative agenda
and right-wing congresspersons in league with fundamentalist
religions and Reverend Jerry Falwell. Terry was gay, he lived
with a lover, he even had an affair with one of my friends; he
was a frequent visitor to the New York disco, bathhouse, and
Fire Island scenes; he moved comfortably in the Washington

gay political community because he knew they would not expose his homosexuality—even as he raised millions of dollars for the enemies of gay people. When a book came out, *God's Bullies* by Perry Deane Young, in which Dolan's homosexuality was revealed, his "heterosexuality" was defended by no less a voice than William Safire, who, in his regular column in *The New York Times*, sharply criticized Young, or anyone, for using such "lies" to discredit Dolan, or any prominent person, and his work. When gays attempted to get a rebuttal to Safire printed in the *Times*, and, when the *Times* refused, in the *Washington Post*, it was not possible to do so. At a gay cocktail party in Washington, I confronted Terry and condemned him for taking so much from our community and repaying us in such a monstrous fashion. I did not expect to be congratulated by the others in attendance, but I certainly did not expect to be condemned by them, which is just what happened. In Washington, one does not criticize one's enemies, even if they are one's own. When Dolan died, from AIDS, his brother, who is a speechwriter in the Reagan White House, attempted to suppress an article that appeared in *Regardies* magazine by *Wall Street Journal* staff writer Ellen Hume, which contained the truth about both his brother's homosexuality and his death from AIDS.

Eight years into an epidemic that has gone largely untended because it is perceived as happening to gays, *and* because gays have not sufficiently demanded the attention it deserves, we witness the tragic spectacle of many tens of thousands dead and many millions infected. It is hard to escape the fact that we gays are helping to kill off our future by protecting this rule of silence. It becomes increasingly difficult, and morally impossible, to sit by silently and watch elected officials (not to mention prominent church leaders) across the nation, whom we know to be closeted gay men or lesbians, as they not only deny their heritage but bend over backwards *not* to help in gay emergencies, lest this very aid, by extension, identify them.

The closeted are also protected by the media and the press, even though it is not against any law to name anyone as gay if that person is gay, if that person has disclosed it publicly, or, as is most important in the case of public officials, if their work in the public arena is compromised by their denying their homosexuality. Terry Dolan would have been a particularly good example of this, should any reporter (other than Young) have had the courage to write his story honestly while Dolan was still alive. But reporters don't discuss a person's homosexuality, not because they or their papers are afraid of lawsuits (which are rarely brought), but because they are worried about offending sources or making themselves personae non gratae.

Representative Barney Frank of Massachusetts, before he came out publicly, had for some time acknowledged privately to many reporters that he was gay; but reporters didn't report it because they thought that he would be offended. If they had reported it, they could not have been sued because (1) it was true, and (2) he regularly debated gay issues publicly. Therefore his sexuality would have been relevant to public understanding of his participation in the debate. As I said, it is no secret to many gays that many of the most important politicians and government bureaucrats forced into dealing with AIDS are doing their work badly, if at all, because they are in the closet, and we cannot get the press to help us expose them.

The battle days of libel cases just for naming a person homosexual are largely gone. That was the legal world that destroyed Oscar Wilde, and it existed until about 1970, when the first mainstream debates in society about homosexuality and the gay rights movement also commenced. Saying someone is gay who *is* gay no longer constitutes defamation or slander or libel. You cannot defame someone by telling the truth. But the press has not caught on or caught up.

So it still comes back to the point that homosexuality is considered something negative. The many of us who are so proud of homosexuality are at the mercy of the many more who aren't. And the law still does protect closeted gays who aren't in the position of politicians or church leaders dealing with gay issues. To name a movie star as gay, even if he or she is (unless he or she debated gay issues), is considered an invasion of privacy. The law doesn't protect Jews denying their Jewishness. Could one imagine the gay actor-playwright Harvey Fierstein getting away with suing someone because he was called a heterosexual?

Homosexuals always seem to be considered entirely as artistic. It comes as a surprise to find Arendt writing, in her essay,

"The Jew as Pariah": "When it comes to claiming its own in the field of European arts and letters, the attitude of the Jewish people may best be described as one of reckless magnanimity. With a grand gesture and without a murmur of protest it has calmly allowed the credit for its great writers and artists to go to other peoples, itself receiving in return (in punctilious regular payments) the doubtful privilege of being acclaimed father of every notorious swindler and mountebank."

It is presently no different for gays. Roy Cohn is identified as gay; John Maynard Keynes is not. Burgess and Maclean are identified as gay; J. Edgar Hoover is not. Boy George is identified as gay; Cole Porter and Lorenz Hart are not.

It appears impossible for homosexuals to claim our own. We "honor" the closetedness of the living. Or we identify our renowned dead, and no journalist, historian, or academic will publish our identification. In the case of the famous dead, like Whitman or Leonardo da Vinci or Michelangelo, some "proof" is required—for everyone since time began is declared heterosexual unless *proved* otherwise. It is not sufficient for us to respond to such questions as "Can you prove he was homosexual?" with our own, "Can you prove he wasn't?" So we are denied our heritage. We are denied the most potent weapons to prove our own worth both to ourselves and to the world.

At the end of his life, Christopher Isherwood urged every homosexual of some authority to reveal his homosexuality. Of all the major widely published poets over fifty, only Allen Ginsberg, Richard Howard, and James Merrill have done so. There can't be just three major gay poets over fifty.

IV

Homosexuals are at an historic moment in our own emergence, and we have been so placed, I would estimate, for ten to fifteen years. When I was a child, I thought I was the only homosexual in the world. When I was a student at Yale, I thought I was one of only a few. Now I have concrete and visible confirmation that I am one of tens of millions, one in eight, one in ten, one of twenty-four million—whichever estimate, they are all comforting. We are here, and seen to be here, and known to be here, more than ever. Beginning with the mid-1970s, much to our surprise and gratification, mental, spiritual, and sexual, we began to take full note of this.

As gays become more visible, we provoke more hatred. As I said, we have, in many cases, comfortable disposable incomes that allow us to live well and deny ourselves little in the way of consumer goods. (Of course, there are poor gays, but, whatever our income, we often have little to spend it on but ourselves.) We have, in most cases, no responsibilities raising children. If we find old houses in marginal neighborhoods and remodel them, thus revitalizing that neighborhood, we're a threat to those living there already. We appear as leeches: taking much from the world but putting little back into it (always excepting our taxes, conveniently overlooked by our critics; and we have historically asked little in return for these annual contributions), though when we try to do so, we are hated even more for our very attempts and visibility. Or our perceived "freedom." My sister-in-law, Alice, once said to me that she was jealous of my life in many ways: I could do what I wanted to do, while her life is circumscribed by a large suburban estate, partnering a successful lawyer in his social and professional endeavors (which are more than a little intertwined), raising and instructing three children in the ways of their world, with little time for herself, while I have nothing but time for myself.

Like Jews, homosexuals historically have had little interest in power. We never think of exercising it, or indeed that we possess it. Of course, this comes from centuries of having no political experience, even though these centuries were eons of tension, ostracism, and, quite often, extermination because we were what we are. We have failed to notice that these centuries also allowed us, as they still do, great possibilities for the use of power, so large are our numbers, as they have always been.

If a reporter wished a quote on women's rights, or the black reaction to anything, the reporter would have at his fingertips a list of many prominent respondents, most of whom have national recognition. One thinks immediately of Gloria Steinem or Betty Friedan, or Jesse Jackson or Barbara Jordan. In all of gay history, there has never been a gay name with national recognition, not at least while he or she was alive.

Why has it been impossible for the huge numbers of homosexuals, in this country and this world, to foster, nurture, and produce such visible leadership?

There are practical reasons: There's no money to be made as a gay leader—it doesn't lead to election to political office anywhere; it doesn't provide a substantial living, because few are the organizations to run and even lower their budgets to pay anyone; nor is it necessarily good for business, unlike, say, being a politician in New York, which has recently enabled so many to make so much. It only leads to aggravation, and eventually to desperation and futility—not only for these reasons, but also because the gay population itself has thus far evinced little interest in participating in what few gay political organizations there are.

The few gay men and lesbians actively involved in the political process, in their so far unsuccessful attempts to make their words heard, thus find themselves scrambling for the few constituents and meager territory available. This has given rise not to cooperation among themselves, but to distrust, anger, and backbiting. Few are able to withstand the toil and anguish of this fighting; the frustrating disillusionment, when realization finally dawns that their inspiration has not been sufficient to attract a crowd and exhaustion sets in, has robbed us of many important voices. The average length of time a person is able to step forth with the best of intentions before being struck down by lassitude or fury seems to be a few years at the most. (San Francisco Supervisor Harvey Milk, the first openly gay person ever elected to public office, was assassinated.)

Any leader not only has to have a message—certainly not hard to come up with—but he or she has to have the ability to raise funds and attract enough supporters. No openly gay leader working for a gay organization has been successful at these tasks, nationally, or for very long.

The National Gay and Lesbian Task Force has a mailing list of 13,000 members. The Human Rights Campaign Fund mails to 22,000. National Gay Rights Advocates mails to 18,000. Lambda Legal Defense and Education fund has 15,000. And a large proportion of these members are the same—i.e., many of us belong to two or more of these organizations. With a potential 24 million joiners, plus supportive friends and families, and with the AIDS crisis threatening us more each day, these are our *largest* political organizations. (We seem able only to summon large numbers to march in parades, which, of course, provide protection for anonymity.) The gay community has nothing like a National Organization of Women, a B'nai B'rith, an NAACP. Even Gay Men's Health Crisis, headquartered in the city worst afflicted with AIDS, and with an estimated one million gay people to draw from, has been able to attract only 1,800 volunteers, a number of them heterosexual women. Sixty-eight percent of GMHC's charitable donations come from heterosexual donors. This is an even more remarkable fact to contemplate when it is realized that 80 percent of GMHC's $12 million total annual budget comes from charitable donations. So much for the perception of successful AIDS fundraising from gays.

Though we lack charismatic leaders with national recognition, we have a superabundance of part-time leaders, dropping in and out of running organizations, depending on their energy and the organization's health. Unfortunately, as in any community where there are many scrambling for the same dollar and the same constituents, there is much territorial infighting— with little realization that there's enough for all if only cooperation and alliances could be forged. Gay organizations in every major city seem eventually to fall victim to endemic bitchiness and bitterness. The very sarcasm that makes gay humor so amusing is also the potent weapon that stabs us to death. And people who should plug into these organizations don't: lawyers, accountants, teachers, doctors; at a time of national emergency it's the professional skills that are needed most.

The backbiting and backstabbing are horrendous, and perhaps typical of most marginal political groups, particularly those on the left—all fighting each other and not the issue, and all being politically ineffective.

When a population cannot even prevent scurrilous attacks on it from appearing in the press, how could it ever mobilize against something like AIDS? A recent issue of *New York Woman* contained comments from the columnist Jimmy Breslin about *Burn This*, a Broadway play by the gay writer Lanford Wilson. "I thought the play was written by a faggot, it's a fag play written for fags. . . . Faggoty—oh, they love fag plays. Anything with latent homosexuality scores big, because that's the strain in this city. You have little unmarried guys building big buildings." That a major New York columnist, late of the *News* and now of *Newsday*, would say anything like this in print, and that a publication would then publish it, shows the extent of our weakness. What paper would publish a description of *Fences* as "a nigger play written for niggers"? Or of *A Shayna Maidel* as "a kike play written for kikes"? Or what newspaper would ask anti-Semites their opinions of a Jewish parade down Fifth Avenue, or note the words on placards racists were holding on the sidelines of a black march, as the *Times* felt compelled to include vicious anti-gay slogans purveyed by no more than twelve along a parade of over 100,000 on Gay Pride Day?

I recently spoke with Vivian Shapiro, the former co-chair of Human Rights Campaign Fund, which, in an era of the declining importance of PACs, is now America's ninth largest one. (HRCF made contributions to the campaigns of politicians they deemed helpful and friendly toward gay issues; unfortunately, a number of the candidates found it embarrassing to receive this money, so concentration has now been turned toward funding several full-time lobbyists in Washington. The entire gay population supports only six lobbyists.) Vivian is popular, an excellent speaker, and an effective fundraiser. After four years of intense political activism, which found her constantly traveling back and forth across the country, to the detriment of her job (she is vice-president of a successful firm that represents major metropolitan newspapers and sells advertising space for them), Shapiro suddenly quit gay politics. "You've got to be a lunatic to volunteer to do this. You lose your personal life. You're exhausted. If you care, you're worried all the time. You don't sleep. You wake up in the middle of the night—until one day you wake up and ask yourself, 'Why am I one of only so few doing this?' And you finally quit in guilt and grief."

This situation repeated that of an earlier promising gay leader, Virginia Apuzzo, who headed the National Gay and Lesbian Task Force for three years. One of the most inspirational speakers in the memories of many, she was unable either to build her membership or to attract donations substantial enough to retire an ever-increasing debt. Finally, one day she left to take a position working in Consumer Affairs for Governor Cuomo.

"Nobody knows what to do anymore," Shapiro says. "I used to think I knew. I just don't know now. I can't personally force 24 million people to come out of the closet."

For a while, San Francisco was the gays' Israel. For decades, gays migrated there, and in time they attained great power in the political structure of that city. No mayor there would consider *not* consulting with gay leaders. And this gay power was sufficient to keep most local heterosexual opposition in check. Tragically, with the devastation of AIDS, gay power in San Francisco has waned considerably: Many of the leaders have died.

Where do we go? We don't have Zionism as a hopeful haven from the world's hatred of us. And, as Arendt pointed out, Zionism's solution was not one of fighting anti-Semitism on its own ground, that is, wherever it existed, but to escape it, "denying the Jewish part of responsibility for existing conditions" in the first place, and sinking "to the assumption, as arbitrary as it is absurd, that every Gentile living with Jews must become a conscious or subconscious Jew-hater." "The upbuilding of Palestine has little to do with answering the anti-Semites; at most it has 'answered' the secret self-hatred and lack of self-confidence on the part of those Jews who have themselves consciously or unconsciously succumbed to some parts of anti-Semitic propaganda." Perhaps homosexuals should be grateful that we're relieved from setting up our own nation-state, though the relief from such an affiliation obliges us to an even sterner battle.

It is, of course, this battle that I think we are losing.

"Every pariah," Arendt declares, "who refused to be a rebel was partly responsible for his own position and therewith for the blot on mankind which it represented. From such shame there was no escape. . . . For insofar as man is more than a mere creature of nature, more than a mere product of Divine creativity, insofar will he be called to account for the things which men do to men in the world which they themselves condition."

Are we at just such a juncture in the development of homosexual emergence into political stability and power? As I mentioned, this notion that every closeted gay person is the single most important hindrance to the achievement of this goal by those out of the closet is something said so often that it has become meaningless. The words, the plea, continue to remain insufficiently inspiring. The gay writer Edmund White, in mock despair, once announced that of the 24 million gays that are supposed to inhabit America, no more than 100,000 were openly so and no more than five thousand of these were politically active.

My friend Robert Prager wrote me from San Diego: "But what is the correct course of action in the world where the worst has happened and is happening?" This is not such a peculiar question as it sounds when one is asking gays to engage in civil disobedience *against* someone. That "someone" quite often receives sympathy for the "persecution" he's receiving at the hands of the hated homos. A candidate who might in fact be sympathetic to gay causes will arrange to be picketed by gays so that he will appeal to the homophobic vote. Rumors of just this sort of strategy on the part of Governor Michael Dukakis have been reported in the gay press. "Oh, I can't vote for homosexuals, a homosexual issue. I'll get killed at home if I vote for those homosexuals": These are the words that liberal Senator Tom Harkin (D.-Iowa) used to chide his fellow senators for their bigotry, hoping to get them to vote against an amendment that would remove an antidiscrimination (against gays) clause from a D.C. ordinance (the Georgetown University case mentioned earlier). The amendment passed overwhelmingly.

In his book, Professor Kateb describes what Hannah Arendt most prized: "Freedom exists only when citizens engage in political action. . . . Arendt's mission as a philosopher is to attempt the recovery of the idea of political action in a culture that she thinks has (except episodically) lost the practice of it and in which almost all philosophy is united, if in nothing else, in denying intrinsic value to it."

The word "political" has, for most gay people, uncomfortable innuendos and repercussions. It suggests we must be obstreperous, obnoxious, rebellious—and visible. We must confront a system that does not want to accept us. For most gay people, the recent decades, even the present one—providing we are not ill with AIDS ourselves; and most gay people mercifully still fall within this category—have been good ones. There appears to be a margin of acceptance, and tolerance enough; no one is yet coming to haul us, as a group, into the streets or march us off to camps. This is comfort enough for most. For those with financial capital, the Reagan years have been generous, and gays, like most people, vote their pocketbooks. Better to accept this existence, most feel, than to make waves and endanger it.

It is overwhelmingly difficult, almost impossible, to change this way of thinking. It is useless constantly to cite references to the dangers into which this attitude led the European Jews. Gays do not identify with Jews, any more than Jews identify with gays. And most Americans, certainly, believe that we've all arrived at a more tolerant time in history, that Santayana's lesson has been learned, and that we can't go back again. To suggest that we most assuredly can is considered, by many gays, ridiculous hyperbole.

In the same way that the creation of Israel was an attempt by the Jews to take control of their lives—and by so doing actually withdrawing themselves from those geographical-political areas where they were most hated, while still thinking that they were doing no such thing, so the institution, growth, and proliferation of myriad AIDS organizations has been considered by many gays as a conscious, positive, creative political response, indeed a historic one, to fight against oppression. Only now do we realize, too late, as did the Jews, that the powerlessness remains. I don't know how many of the hundreds of volunteers to GMHC and its fellow satellites across the country actually thought, when signing up, that they could help change the course of this epidemic "politically," a word as much anathema to them as it was to millions of Jews before the war, but I'm certain they considered this contribution of their time and energy as a step in this direction—certainly a more "political" act than most of them had ever participated in for any gay cause in their pasts. I believe that for most of them there was some sort of inchoate, unverbalized, perhaps even unconscious, but nevertheless existing notion inside them that, somewhere, there were leaders, there was leadership—somewhere in the hierarchy of the organization, with its board of directors and honorary directors and numerous well-known contributors and supporters—which would be on the front lines, in Washington, or New York City, or Albany, or Sacramento, petitioning for all the requisite materiel for winning the war.

I doubt that it occurred to any of these volunteers that GMHC (and its fellow AIDS organizations across the country) has actually made it easier for the system to ignore gays and AIDS. (Theodor Herzl, the founder of Zionism, once described Jewish charity as "a mechanism for keeping the needy in subjection." This is cited by Ron H. Feldman in his excellent collection of Arendt's miscellaneous writings, *The Jew as Pariah.*) These community self-help organizations have removed a huge burden of responsibility from the local, state, and federal governments. The services they are diligently providing are services these governments *should be providing.* Indeed, contributors are paying twice for these services, the first time in their taxes.

But, people protest, if GMHC et al. didn't provide these services, no one would be providing them. Perhaps. But not providing such services—including crisis counseling; legal, welfare, and ombudsman advisers; group therapies of many sorts; and community education—would long since have shamed an administration into its duty. Obviously some people aren't going to sit by and uncomplainingly let their friends die. But it doesn't seem to register that if you're going to do something yourself to alleviate the problem because your government refuses to, you have to protest *twice* as much against that government inaction. Not complain less, but complain more. As Arendt wrote to support her thesis: "The simple truth is that Jews will have to fight anti-Semitism everywhere or else be exterminated everywhere."

Even with AIDS, where there is an emergency that far surpasses such other gay problems as immigration, adoption, discrimination, anti-gay violence (although these also are endemic to AIDS), the organizations that have been founded discover in very short order that a conservative attitude is the first thing to arrive in the board room as soon as minimal success in numbers and dollars has been achieved. Gone immediately are all the original intentions to fight to make the system accountable. As organizations such as GMHC attract prominent closeted lawyers or wealthy heterosexual socialites, conservatism becomes even more entrenched than when the organization was run by inexperienced, naïve, young gay volunteers, who, at least, had fury on their side and anger as their original agenda.

What has happened, of course, and this applies to all governmental agencies as well, is that energy is being converted to *managing* the crisis, turning the crisis into a condition, something that is a part of the way things are, something that happens like a flood or hurricanes or poverty—to be managed, thus creating new bureaucracies. The very source of the problem is ignored and negated. As Randy Shilts, author of *And the Band Played On*—a book filled with as much damning evidence on AIDS being ignored as Jonathan Kozol's *Rachel and Her Children* is filled with facts on the ignoring of the homeless—said, "AIDS didn't just happen. It was allowed to happen."

All these AIDS organizations are *managing* AIDS. No one is trying to *stop* it. It is impossible now, and has been impossible from the very beginning, to get the ear of our President, our mayor, our governor, any of the Presidential candidates (with the honorable exception of Jesse Jackson), or indeed that of the two most important government officials in charge: Dr. Otis Bowen, the director of the Department of Health and Human Resources, and Dr. James Wyngaarden, the director of the National Institutes of Health, both of whom have been singularly silent on the issue. What Dr. Mathilde Krim, the founding co-chair of the American Foundation for AIDS Research, said from the very beginning must not be forgotten: "This is an epidemic that could have been contained. Everything about this epidemic has been utterly predictable, from the very beginning, from the very first day. But no one would listen. There are many people who knew exactly what was happening, what would happen and has happened, but no one of any importance would listen. They still won't listen. We definitely could have contained it."

It seems not to occur to an organization that has placed the wife of one of New York's wealthiest men, with connections at the White House itself, on its board—as GMHC has so placed Joan Tisch, wife of Preston Tisch, Reagan's former Postmaster General—that the thing to do would be to have this wife or, even better, her husband, deliver a plea to the President. If they are thinking of this possibility, they are not acting on it. I have been unable to understand why Elizabeth Taylor, AmFar's other co-chair, for all her considerable devotion to the AIDS fight, never achieved a personal meeting with Ronald Reagan, certainly someone she knows or has access to as a fellow performer, if nothing else. Such a meeting—scheduled as it would be with a list of requests, and publicized as it should be to let the world know whether it was granted or not—would do far greater good than hours of fundraising in Miami Beach.

Gays are certainly not alone in disdaining political action. Arendt, in *The Human Condition,* traces this disparagement all the way back to an early and continuing fundamental doctrine of the Christian faith—a faith that insists on the possibility of eternal life, which "brought hope to those who knew that their world was doomed, indeed a hope beyond hope, since the new message promised an immortality they never had dared to hope for. This reversal could not but be disastrous for the esteem and the dignity of politics." Kateb says, "The desire to substitute the inner life for a worldly life is understandable, but for Arendt unforgivable." This same desire is no doubt partly responsible for many of the noble deeds of sacrifice offered up by countless volunteers. (It is also no doubt partly responsible for the fatalistic attitude of so many: "If I'm going to go, I'm going to go.")

I don't know if gay people are "more religious" than non-gays. I do think there is such an amazing compliance with the rules of the world, and how it is run, and such an extreme avoidance of upsetting apple carts, as to be traced, less to centuries of religion, than to childhoods of being raised as good little boys and girls, obedient to parents and school and church. We knew we were different, and we knew we were hateful to institutions, and this resulted only in our denying our naturalness, not in our confronting the institutions that hated us. Gay children will often attempt suicide rather than tell their parents about their homosexuality; "I don't want to hurt them" is the unvarying answer in response to "Why don't you tell them you're gay?" The response that is never made is, "Haven't my parents hurt me by hating homosexuality?" "I love you, dear, even if you're gay" seems to be the most supportive parental acknowledgment most honest gay children can hope for. For too many gays with AIDS, their parents would rather have them *die* than admit they're gay. (There are too many cases of gay sons going home to die, to be with parents and family who haven't known these sons were gay or had AIDS; and, when confronted with both these facts, these parents and these families turned these sons out.)

For Arendt, there is no higher calling than the political. "The *raison d'être* of politics is freedom, and its field of experience is action." *(Between Past and Future.)* Arendt drew her inspiration from ancient Greece (for gay people, also that last page in history when we were free and accepted), where all citizens were willing to participate in the political process. For Arendt political action was a moral imperative. She even thought that civil disobedience was permissible, and that any democracy must allow it. She was very much in favor of the civil rights and antiwar movements, so anchored in demonstrations. Professor Kateb collects her thoughts: "In modern times the civil disobedients are precisely those who guard the limits on the conduct of office-holders. . . . When those in authority attack the Constitution, *and* when judicial review is denied [both certainly applicable in the gay community, particularly since the recent *Bowers v. Hardwick* case in which the Supreme Court ruled against the legality of consenting homosexual acts in the privacy of one's own home], citizens may apply irregular pressures, including lawbreaking, to defend it." The important thing is to get the government not to welch on its constitutional promises.

V

Perhaps this is a good place to say why Hannah Arendt interests me so. I'm old enough to remember vividly the deafening roars of outrage that greeted her "Eichmann in Jerusalem: A Report on the Banality of Evil," which she wrote in 1963 on assignment for *The New Yorker,* and which has remained in print, and blanketed in imbroglio, ever since. Most of the outrage, it would appear, erupted, and continues to fester, because

of an imprecise reading of her intentions, even though, as
Arendt's biographer, Elisabeth Young-Bruehl (in *Hannah
Arendt: For Love of the World*) says, "Arendt's book did lend
itself to misinterpretation more than any other she wrote: its
conclusions were shocking, it contained numerous small errors
of fact, it was often ironic in style and imperious in tone, and
some of its most controversial passages were peculiarly insensitive."

The particular "controversy" that upset so many Jews, and
which I admire her hugely for having the guts to raise, was the
question of the Jews' own complicity in their mass extermination. The imprecision of her antagonists' reading based itself on
a belief that she had said Jews let themselves be marched off
to death. "I never asked why the Jews 'let themselves be
killed,' " Arendt wrote in her defense, in a letter to her old
friend Gershom Scholem (included in *The Jew as Pariah*). "On
the contrary, I accused Hausner [the prosecuting attorney in
the Eichmann case] of having posed this question to witness
after witness. There was no people and no group in Europe
which reacted differently under the immediate pressure of terror. The question I raised was that of the cooperation of Jewish
functionaries during the 'Final Solution' . . . I said that there
was no possibility of resistance [at this late date in events], but
there existed the possibility of *doing nothing.*"

Arendt felt it was these functionaries—prominent members
of Jewish communities—who, under the supremely misguided
notion that they were staving off Jewish deaths by performing,
unfortunately superbly, all the necessary administrative duties
the Nazis requested of them, actually brought these deaths
closer to reality. Had these Jewish functionaries refused to
cooperate, had everyone in essence refused to do anything but
be passive, the Nazis, with far fewer numbers, would have been
unable to kill so *many* millions. But "wherever Jews lived,
there were recognized Jewish leaders, and this leadership, almost without exception, cooperated in one way or another, for
one reason or another, with the Nazis."

Like Arendt, I believe that my people must answer for a
large part of our current predicament. Despite what the Constitution says, one usually has a hard time obtaining one's constitutional rights unless a concerted demand is made for them. If

one is poor, black, and uneducated, there are very good reasons why fighting is difficult. If one is economically comfortable, gay, and educated, these reasons evaporate. Like Arendt, "I can admit to you something beyond that, namely, that wrong done by my own people naturally grieves me more than wrong done by other peoples." Twenty-four million men and women sitting silently by as the AIDS epidemic continues to gobble up their own is wrong. The world is what we make of it: This is the cornerstone of Arendtian thinking. I don't believe that we made AIDS, but I believe, by our not rising up in any coherent, cohesive, visible way, we allow it to continue. Jews aren't less responsible, or, in Arendt's words, don't "cease to be coresponsible," because they're victims "of the world's injustice and cruelty." Too many gay people hide behind the mother's apron of "the world's injustice and cruelty." It's easier that way. It's easier and simpler to be a victim than a fighter. If homosexuals are so politically blind that we don't understand the implications of our own actions (and inactions), then we must pay yet a further price. One is responsible for the human world, Arendt said, even if one is a victim.

In her essay, "Organized Guilt and Universal Responsibility," written in 1945, Arendt wrote: "It is many years now that we meet Germans who declare that they are ashamed of being Germans. I have often felt tempted to answer that I am ashamed of being human."

The lessons the Jews eventually learned when their own numbers were threatened and destroyed are the lessons all homosexuals avoid studying at our peril.

VI

"It is no mere accident," Arendt wrote in "The Moral of History," "that the catastrophic defeats of the peoples of Europe began with the catastrophe of the Jewish people, a people in whose destiny all others thought they could remain uninterested."

It's not too early to see AIDS as the homosexuals' holocaust. I have come reluctantly to believe that genocide is occurring: that we are witnessing—or *not* witnessing—the
systematic, planned annihilation of some by others with the
avowed purpose of eradicating an undesirable portion of the
population.

I know that straight Jews, and other heterosexuals, find this
comparison of holocausts repugnant.

I certainly don't know what it was like to witness six million
die. When I say that I have lost some five hundred acquaintances and friends over the past seven years, I have been told
point-blank by straight Jewish people that "their" extermination is the only "holy" one; ours, by contrast, is piddling. Evidently I must not get so upset, because my deaths are less than
their deaths.

Does it appear that I am intentionally trying to escalate our
horror to that of the Supreme Horror? I am not unfamiliar with
charges of hysteria and hyperbole. To read Primo Levi is to
know that our suffering, as of this moment, is still small in
comparison. But Primo Levi also writes, "A certain dose of
rhetoric is perhaps indispensable for memory to persist."

One inadvertent fallout from *the* Holocaust is the growing
inability to view any other similar tragedies as awful. Jews
themselves are partly responsible for this: memory must in no
way be tampered with. But, important as this memory is, the
insistence on its primogeniture frustrates efforts to arouse
equal public concern when the newest children on the block
arrive, demanding immediate succor.

What Hannah Arendt was trying to tell the Jews was that,
whether they knew it or not, they have been able to survive thus
far because, like it or not, they constituted a political community, and if they wanted to survive they had to break, as Ron
H. Feldman puts it in his introduction to *The Jew as Pariah*,
"with the past in which accident reigned supreme and take
conscious control of their destiny."

The years Arendt writes about were ones in which "being
a Jew does not give any legal status in the world." It is hard
for young Jews to remember this time, and it is hard for gays
to believe Jews were once as unrecognized as gays are now.

Gays remain pretty unconvinced when told that it took World War II to organize the Jewish population finally and effectively—those of them who were left.

(Because I am also Jewish, and find so many similarities in the historic plights of both Jews and gays, I find it painful that my religion is, in most instances, so unkind, uncharitable, and in some instances—that of the Orthodox and Hasidim—downright murderous. People, if they learn lessons at all, learn them, it would appear, only for themselves, and then only if they are lucky. The benefits are evidently neither transferable generally or assignable specifically.)

"The realization that millions of Jews had gone to their deaths without resistance resulted in a change in Jewish consciousness," Feldman writes, then quoting Arendt: "Gone, probably forever, is that chief concern of the Jewish people for centuries: survival at any price. Instead, we find something essentially new among Jews, the desire for dignity at any price."

This longing for dignity at any price has overtaken the gay population in the largest cities. Our holocaust has done that for us. We have learned, if not how to fight, or become "political," how to grieve magnificently. We have established organizations, many of them now huge and rich, to cater to the dying. It is almost as if, rather than bother anyone with our problems, certainly rather than fight to correct what caused them, we shall clutch them possessively to our bosoms and suffer as nobly as we can. It is indeed heroic to witness the amazing devotion that so many, gay and straight, lavish on their dying friends. I do not mean to diminish these sad rituals, though indeed I personally find them slightly ghoulish.

Of course I want to be attended to by those I love when my time comes. I am just slightly stunned when I witness so many electing to give such large amounts of energy, devotion, and caring to these morbid activities, rather than attempting to right the wrongs in a system that's made these activities necessary in the first place. I look at faces at countless memorial services and cannot comprehend why the connection isn't made between these deaths and going out to fight so that more of these deaths, including possibly one's own, can be staved off. Huge numbers regularly show up in cities for Candlelight

Marches, all duly recorded for the television cameras. Where are these same numbers when it comes to joining political organizations, with either their dollars or their skills, or plugging in to the incipient civil disobedience movement represented in ACT UP?

I find in these actions a defeatism that is depressingly negative: Gays are hated, these actions seem to say, and there's nothing to be done about it, gays will always be hated, so let's accept this as we bury our dead.

That an increasingly large number of these saints—and I do think there's also a margin of saintliness inherent here, as well as a yearning for such saintliness—are straight women I find both disturbing and gratifying. But it's as if, not only do we tell ourselves that fighting for our lives is a useless occupation, but now we are joined by heterosexual representatives telling us the same thing and helping us to nail our coffins.

I submit that there are different kinds of holocausts. After all, the word is defined, in my *American Heritage Dictionary*, as "any widespread destruction." Hitler gave it new and grotesque meaning, but despite the Jewish insistence that the word is now totally attached to their own destruction, it is perversely inhuman to deny its attachment to other conflagrations. At this moment in history, it is perhaps thought that such a holocaust as Hitler perpetrated can never happen again, and Jews fight mightily to keep this notion alive, even though there certainly have been mighty holocausts since: Stalin's and Ethiopia's, as well as incomprehensible slaughters in Biafra, Cambodia, and Lebanon, are only the few that come immediately to mind. The Jewish outrage that automatically erupts whenever another endangered minority, under threat of destruction, claims that a holocaust is occurring is selfishly counterproductive to confronting yet another example of man's seemingly innate inhumanity to man.

Certainly, a holocaust does not require a Hitler to be effective. Certainly, a holocaust does not require *deliberate* intentionality on the part of one or several or many or a bureaucracy to be effective. Holocausts can occur, and probably most often do occur, because of *inaction*. This inaction can be unintentional or deliberate. How one defines the line, or level, of intentionality or unintentionality is often a difficult question. How does one accuse a bureaucrat of looking the other way, or of paying no attention, or of paying less attention than he should, when he can counter—as Adolf Eichmann did—with the defense, "I was only doing my job as best I could"?

In all my investigations over these past years into why AIDS has not been attended to with the dispatch it warrants, I have been told at almost every juncture that "all is being done that can be done." Indeed, I'm often accused of being "ungrateful" for this "activity," and that more has been learned about this condition in a shorter time than in any other health emergency. To this hyperbole, I usually add my own: If AIDS were happening to Jews, or to American Legionnaires, or to white tennis players at country clubs, we would be much farther along the road to treatment and cure than we are, which, despite all protestations to the contrary, is not very far at all.

The one facet of the AIDS epidemic that I think almost everyone prefers to overlook is this: *Something infectious is going around.* Whatever the cause (and, as I have said, and it bears repeating, like almost everything connected with this epidemic, I tend to view any statement of definite fact with doubt, so many have been contradicted, contravened, or proved downright wrong since these statements of "fact" started appearing in 1981), it is apparently being transmitted infectiously, and it is not stopping. Nothing has changed since the onset about the most important prediction: There may never be a cure. As Dr. Linda Laubenstein, a hematologist at New York University Medical Center and one of the first doctors to note AIDS in patients and to this day one of the leading doctors treating it, says, "We don't have a very good record of dealing with viruses. There isn't a virus yet that's been cured or eliminated. The best we can hope for, and this is a long way from ever happening, is that there will be some kind of treatment that will be suppressive without being too toxic to use over a lifetime—the way diabetics take insulin."

Opponents of increased AIDS funding use, as one of their excuses, the high fatalities from other horrors, such as lung cancer, various lymphomas, heart disease, even auto accidents. These, they say, are just as much in need of attention. "But they're not infectious," is Dr. Laubenstein's curt response to this kind of thinking.

If I harp on my holocaust comparisons, it is because it is my firm belief that we are in but the early stages of destruction by AIDS of huge swaths of the world's population. And the hideously alarming World Health Organization figures don't seem to do the trick of convincing any powers-that-be. There have been, over these past three years, four damning reports prepared for President Reagan or at his behest: two by the National Academy of Sciences, one by his Surgeon General, Dr. C. Everett Koop, and one, most recently, by his own Presidential Commission on the Human Immunodeficiency Virus Epidemic. Each has said more or less the same thing. The leading editorial in the Sunday *New York Times* of June 5th, 1988, congratulating the commission for its "findings," noted (in words that could as justifiably be applied to the *Times* itself): "The Administration's response to AIDS has from the start been torpid, fitful, fragmented and riven with prejudice against those infected with the virus." The Commission's Report itself says that government leadership "has been inconsistent and not properly coordinated"; the federal response has been "slow, halting, and uneven"; the Food and Drug Administration and the National Institutes of Health were particularly criticized for going *very* slowly indeed.

Amazingly enough, it is no longer even a question of money. Over very long years, Congress has gradually increased its appropriations, so that now there appears to be enough to go around. What Congress is now finding is that this money isn't being spent, or is being spent unwisely, and that no one is in charge of supervising its proper allocation. To cite just one heinous example of malfeasance, Dr. Anthony Fauci, the director of the National Institute for Allergy and Infectious Diseases—that branch of the NIH under which most AIDS treatment research falls—was recently raked over the coals, first at hearings conducted by Representative Ted Weiss and his House Subcommittee on Human Resources, and subsequently by Senator Edward Kennedy, at Senate hearings conducted by his Committee on Labor and Human Resources, who accused Fauci of "doubletalk." Dr. Fauci has had at his disposal some $374 million. He has been unable to set up a network of hospital treatment centers around the country to test, quickly, promising new drugs (calculated, as I mentioned, to be some two hundred by medical reporter Susan Spencer on "CBS Evening News," and most of them unavailable legally in this country until they *are* tested by the NIH and approved by the FDA). After two years, not only is this system not functioning in any coherent way, but 80 percent of the studies Dr. Fauci and one of his many, many committees, and subcommittees, have approved are still only with AZT, a problematic drug that, in any case, has *already* been approved by the FDA. Because of the snail-like pace of Dr. Fauci's work, and because of the equal lethargy of response from the FDA, which must license any treatment that is approved (and certainly because of the lack of effective pressure from gays or AIDS organizations like GMHC), most of these two hundred untested drugs must be obtained by sufferers as best they can. Hence these treatments are unavailable to any but the rich or the most persistently cagy. Dr. Fauci has been described as "a bumbler" by one of the members of the President's AIDS Commission. I myself have called him, in print, an incompetent idiot.

It is not possible to condemn the stupidities of the NIH without adding those of the FDA. They are a dog-and-pony show. The system is such that you can't have one without the other. A drug tested at the NIH must still be approved by the FDA. Dr. Fauci's culpabilities are equal in size to those of Dr. Frank Young, the FDA's director. Despite repeated promises, despite pressure from congressional subcommittees, presidential reports, and even from Vice-President Bush himself, Dr. Young has done nothing to lessen the eight to nine years' time required for a drug to wend its way leisurely through the FDA approval process. (The average length of time AIDS patients have to live is five years.) Dr. Young loudly trumpeted some new regulations about a year ago—ones that would allow drugs that showed promising efficacy to be available to American patients; but in practice he and his staff have demanded *proof* of this efficacy, not just promise of it, and the time required for that proof to be proved to the FDA is eight to nine years.

A particularly inhumane example of what *is* going on scientifically involves an NIH-sponsored study to test the effectiveness of intravenous immune globulin (an existing pharmaceutical product that anyone can get) on four hundred

babies with AIDS or ARC. These babies have an average age
of eighteen months to two years. Almost all of them are black
or Hispanic. It takes four to eight hours for each intravenous
infusion. An infusion is administered once every twenty-eight
days, for a period of two years. Previous research has revealed
that a high number of the babies have to be *physically restrained* during the infusion. Half of the babies will receive a
useless placebo. Even those babies receiving placebos must be
hooked up to an IV and restrained; because it is assumed that
many of the babies will pick up typical hospital infections, the
NIH wants to make sure these infections are equally distributed among those receiving both placebo and the actual
drug. As if this type of enforced experimentalization was not
cruel enough, and as if making half the babies receive a placebo
under the same circumstances was not cruel enough, it turns
out that it was not necessary to use placebos at all. There
already are in existence earlier results to utilize for statistical
comparisons. When these earlier studies were presented to the
NIH, studies that would save two hundred babies from a need-
less and painful ordeal, the NIH elected to proceed with the
study nevertheless.

The Presidential Commission Report, its strong condemna-
tions and recommendations—they are all words gay men have
longed to hear. But, as I said, we've heard them all before, in
those three earlier reports, which produced as little result as,
in our despondency, we expect this new report to duplicate.
There is no gay man who believes that anything helpful will
actually be accomplished while President Reagan is in office.
(Or if George Bush is elected.) His Commission's Report is seen
as window dressing, perfectly timed so that he doesn't have to
do anything, for he'll be out of office shortly after its receipt.
Again, with the exception of Jesse Jackson, not one of the many
candidates who recently competed for their party's nomination
mentioned AIDS, dealt with AIDS, addressed any AIDS issues,
or presented a plan for the future—a future that, without any
doubt, is going to burden any administration with mountainous
problems far surpassing any of the ones these candidates *are*
willing to discuss. They know that AIDS is not a topic the
electorate wishes to hear about. And no one ever seems to ask,
nor does any of these four reports address the questions: Just

why is it so many people take drugs? Just why is it so many gay
men were promiscuous? Just why is it so many people are
homeless?

If it is not possible to locate one Hitler responsible for allowing this AIDS destruction to multiply so, it is possible to locate
a number of junior candidates. "We don't have one Hitler," a
friend of mine said; "we have many Mengeles."

Ronald Reagan, Dr. Bowen, Dr. Wyngaarden, doctors at the
NIH and FDA, are equal to Hitler and his Nazi doctors performing their murderous experiments in the camps—not because of similar intentions, but because of similar results.

"You either wait while six million again die, which is complicity, or you do something about it. It is just as sinful to let
people die as to gas them." This was said by my best friend,
Rodger McFarlane, who then went on to recite to me sentences
from Christian theology—about sins of commission and omis-
sion—from a religion he no longer believes in.

With all due respect, it doesn't appear piddling to me to
place my five hundred dead friends on the altar of history, and
to posit the possibility that, at the rate we are going, we are now
in a situation historically equivalent to, say, the German Jews
circa 1938–1940, when the looming danger was, for the most
part, also pooh-poohed. And that there will be millions of gay
men dead before our holocaust is over. How can everyone avoid
seeing this? How can straight and gay people continue to deny
the viciousness of the AIDS epidemic? Why do gay men need
to be *convinced* that we are being murdered?

Reluctantly, though for some time I denied this, and fought
against it, for I know it is hugely counterproductive, I have
found myself coming to hate heterosexuals. All heterosexuals.
The ones, naturally, who sit by and ignore or simply observe
what is happening to us. The ones who offer me condolences for
all the awful things happening to us now, as they would in
passing along kind words for a sick friend or relief from a cold
that won't go away. The ones who invite me for Thanksgiving
and Christmas and offer up prayers to God for a surcease to
"Larry's friends who are suffering so much" before commenc-
ing to consume the turkey. The ones who help us bury so many
dead and do not recognize that such deaths need not continue

to occur. I hate them for not doing what I am unable to do—change all this. The same reason they hate me.

The greatest criminal of the century was, to Arendt, the "jobholder and the good family man" who did everything out of "kind concern and earnest concentration on the welfare of his family." "In contrast to the earlier units of the SS men and the Gestapo, Himmler's overall organization relied not on fanatics, nor on congenital murderers, nor on sadists; it relied entirely upon the normality of jobholders and family men."

The family. The family. How these words are repeated and repeated in America—from campaign rhetoric to television commercials. This is a country that prides itself on proclaiming family values, as if there were no others, as if every family was homespun and united and loving, as if it is necessary to produce a child—like a product—to justify or countenance a sexual act. AIDS goes against *all* family values: It is perceived as happening mostly to gay men; it is spread sexually (as if heterosexuals did not have sex); it is an embarrassment. Well, I am a member of a family, too. Or I once thought so. Every gay man has two parents, and other relatives, too. How convenient for them all to have disposed of us so expeditiously, just when we need them most. But the ranks are closed, something is happening to gay men, and we are suddenly no longer affiliated with *the* family. Where do they think we came from? The cabbage patch?

Most gay people see little to admire or to emulate in heterosexual life. It seems filled with hypocrisies we have worked hard to avoid. We see few happy straight marriages and many dishonest ones—husbands and wives cheating on each other, children taking more drugs than we ever took, and people ignoring values that we have made important in our lives: taste, style, education, directness, honesty, energy, friendships. We feel particularly blessed by so many and such strong friendships. We have turned to our friends to take the place of families. "Your friends are your family" is something often heard in conversations of gay people gathered together. We look at Ronald and Nancy Reagan, and the books their own children have written about them, and we watch our President and his wife talk constantly about "family values in America," and we laugh. At least our promiscuity was *honest.*

VII

I spoke earlier about Luke, the appealing man who offered me love. After five dates, I decided not to see him anymore. I offer here a reasonable facsimile of the thoughts that crisscrossed my consciousness while he held me in his arms:

I don't want to die, this is killing me, my need to love can't be worth this—he is so nice, I want him so, he is so gentle and he makes me feel good—he takes me for what I am, and he is kind to me, and he is all the things I have always longed for in a relationship, but my work, my work must come first, I have too much yet to say, I cannot abandon my work, and yet why might it not work out?, why might we not be carriers?, why not take the chance?: But the chance is Russian roulette and the risks are too great, the odds are too much against us, and, too, I might kill him, I might be the carrier, and his life is precious, his youth, he has so much he wants to give to the world. . . .

What it amounts to is that I cannot stand the torture that each coupling brings to our lovemaking, and the nightmares that come into my dreams, and the walking dialogue that plagues me every time I think of it. It constantly jams itself into my thoughts: You must be crazy, you must be out of your mind, you are gambling with your life. Suddenly it doesn't seem to be worth it. When he leaves me, I promise myself I won't see him again. I cannot wait for him to leave. He keeps kissing me goodbye, tenderly, as he goes off to take the GMHC volunteer training—he wants to become a Crisis Counselor, like his sister-in-law, helping to tend the dying. But when he is gone, I miss him already, and I wonder if somehow we can't work it out. No. I must hold firm to my decision. But I miss him. Why didn't I ask him to come back tonight? He has no place to stay before returning to the training tomorrow, without going home to his parents in New Jersey. "Check in," I said, noncommittally, when he left. Will he? When? What will I say then? Do a Nancy Reagan and "Just say no"?

Hours later I am still trying not to think of him. But it's there inside me, my desire for him, my sweet memories, the ingestion of him, symbolic, but perhaps, accidentally, actual. I try to deny these feelings and get to work. Work! I must work. Another hour later, I vomit.

I find I've made this note in my diary after he left, after our fifth night together: When we hold each other, there are three people in bed and one of them is Death. I confide in no one, not even Rodger, who was my former lover and with whom I share everything. In one of our many daily phone conversations, he volunteers, "I think Jesus would have to carry me in his arms to Paris for me to put out."

I am going to say a few words about "gay promiscuity," and let it go. Promiscuity is a loaded word and a controversial subject, and what exactly constitutes promiscuity—how many more than one encounter with how many more than one person?—seems to differ depending on whom you ask. In any event, as Professor Boswell of Yale writes: "There does not seem to be any evidence that gay people are more or less sexual than others." Dr. Richard Isay, a practicing psychoanalyst and Clinical Associate Professor of Psychiatry at Cornell Medical College, writes in his forthcoming book, *Being Homosexual:* "Human males in general are more interested in variations of sexual partners than females." To which Dr. Kinsey's words can be added: "This is the history of his anthropoid ancestors, and this is the history of unrestrained males everywhere." Promiscuity is liberating for some people while for others it's dehumanizing, and thus it's hard to come down on one side or the other without taking into account who's being promiscuous. But the gay community, both before and after the arrival of AIDS, has taken a bad rap for it. The entire heterosexual world, it sometimes seems to me, perceives the entire homosexual world as busily involved in doing nothing but performing endless acts of sexual intercourse. Some of us did and most of us didn't (and now pretty much all of us don't). But it's an issue that must be addressed because if AIDS is transmitted sexually in any way, then there's no question that the promiscuity of some gay men was unwittingly responsible for AIDS killing so many of us. And it's this, of course, that we are being blamed for (particularly by religious groups)—spreading AIDS.

The concept of making a virtue out of sexual freedom, i.e., promiscuity, came about because gay men had nothing else to

call their own *but* their sexuality. The heterosexual majority
has for centuries denied us every possible right of human dignity (which the doctrines of all religions and most "free" countries, as well our own Constitution, are meant to guarantee for
all). The right to marry. The right to tax advantages and employee benefits that married couples enjoy. The right to own
property jointly without fear that the law will disinherit the
surviving partner. The right to hold a job as an openly gay
person. The right to have children. The right not to be discriminated against in just about every area. Indeed—the right
to walk down the street holding hands, as heterosexual people
can do freely when they are in love. The right to love. We are
denied the right to love. Can any heterosexual imagine being
denied the right to love? I ask you to try to imagine how you
might feel if you had to hide from the whole world the fact that
you loved your wife or husband.

So, rightly or wrongly—wrongly, as it turned out—many
gay men decided to make a virtue of the only thing the straight
world didn't have control of: our sexuality. Had we possessed
these rights denied us, had we been allowed to live respectably
in a community of equals, I think a good case could be made
that there would never have been an AIDS epidemic such as we
are seeing. Had we been allowed to marry, many of us would
not have felt the obligation to be promiscuous. (While we may
not see much to emulate in heterosexual marriages, this does
not preclude our desire to try it ourselves. It wouldn't be the
first time we've demonstrated to the straight world that we can
do something better.) Thus I think a good case also can be made
that the AIDS pandemic is the fault of the heterosexual white
majority.

"Our society does not now want gay men to be in stable,
responsible, mutually gratifying relationships," Dr. Isay
writes. "The visibility of such couples is too shattering to the
sense of masculinity of men in most segments of our culture."
Until this change comes—a change that will benefit both gay
men and society alike—the destruction of American homosexuals by the heterosexual majority will continue. It is unrealistic
to think that, even with AIDS, an entire population will be able
to stop having sex. The irony, of course, is that being promiscuous is a characteristic that straight men congratulate each

other on achieving, at the same time they condemn us for the same acts.

The leveling of this blame for the AIDS epidemic is perhaps better understood if an extension of this argument is presented: that the poor, black, and Hispanic have also been forced into AIDS by oppression. The awfulness of their destitution and deprivation, the absolutely zero chance so many of them face in bettering their lot in this world, forces them to seek peaceful respite and brief relief in the only oblivion available to them— the never-never land of drugs. And these drugs, for all the Just Say No mentality of an imbecilic First Lady, this society makes remarkably available through inept law enforcement and just plain looking the other way. It's almost as if a conscious decision had been made somewhere in government to let all these people drug themselves to death.

AIDS having thus been caused to seed and sprout, it was *allowed* to grow and fester and increase a millionfold by the inaction of our government. As I noted earlier, everyone is more interested in *managing* this epidemic than in stopping it, than in taking any time to search for and begin to solve the root causes of what is going on.

VIII

I've perhaps relied too heavily on others' words in trying to state my case. I've done it intentionally. I've been criticized so often and attacked so continuously for so much of my rhetoric that I've tried to find support for my feelings in the philosophies of others whose lives have given them little choice but to think about tragedy and attempt to find, if not definitive explanation, rhyme, or reason, at least a few ground rules on how to get to tomorrow.

I go to many memorial services. I've been to too many where the Bible is invoked, and there are many quotations, like this from the Gospel of John, describing the death of Lazarus: "I am the resurrection and the life; he who believes in me, though he die, yet shall he live, and whoever lives and believes in me shall

never die." Every priest, minister, rabbi, or lay speaker seems
to put forth versions of the same sentiment. It was refreshing,
and quite ennobling, to hear refutation at last. At one service—
that for the writer Michael Grumley—the critic and novelist
Doris Grumbach had this to say: "The Christian in me would
believe in a purpose and a design to life and to the natural
world, but such teleology is very difficult at moments like this.
To wipe out the brightest, most talented, and most beautiful
among us does not seem the action of a just and compassionate
God, a God of love who permits this suffering and these deaths
to happen."

At another service, for my friend Charlie, the minister had
been sent up from the South by Charlie's ex-wife, who hadn't
seen him in twenty years. This minister of God was a fundamentalist, and he was accompanied by Charlie's two daughters,
whom Charlie had supported all their lives, and who somehow
loved him and had been allowed, if not to see him, to talk to him
regularly on the phone. Charlie hadn't consciously known he
was gay when he married and became a father. When he realized he was, he immediately told his wife and she just as immediately divorced him. Now, after all these years, the wife
demanded of Charlie's lover—in return for allowing the daughters to attend—that her minister conduct the memorial service,
a service she herself would not go to. In front of a congregation
composed entirely of Charlie's gay New York friends, this man
began his sermon about sin. Charlie had sinned, and God would
forgive the sinner. Riverside Church was exceptionally quiet.
In nervousness or embarrassment or disgust, men looked at
each other but no one walked out. And then a man got up and
screamed out at the preacher: "Charlie wasn't a sinner. Charlie
was a fine man and as good a father as he was allowed to be.
Charlie wasn't a sinner." And then, obviously surprised at his
own temerity at screaming in a church, he turned and ran out.

I recently got a letter from my old friend and squash partner
Val Cavalier, who now lives in New Orleans. I didn't know he'd
been diagnosed with AIDS. He's terrified, though bravely trying not to be. "I'm tired of candlelight vigils," he wrote to me.
"I think we need blowtorches. And we don't need these so-
called faiths [Val's a Catholic]: beware of priests and suchlike

bearing gifts; they are one of our chief natural enemies. Oh, Larry, it's so scary, this ineffable Fiend I'm dealing with. One of my fellow PWA's [Persons With AIDS] said at a funeral, 'There but for the grace of Gawd.' I said fuck your fuckin' twisted gawd—we/I didn't do *nothin'* to deserve *this.*"

My dear and precious friend, the film historian Vito Russo, sick now three years, gets his energy from being a constant scrapper. He pounds out articles filled with fury, and delivers speeches wherever he can, and he is a constant letter writer to any and all who dare not to understand what we are going through. He is a very busy man. At a sparsely attended ACT UP rally in Albany, in front of those bleak and passionless government buildings on a gray day, he shouted out to those few who trekked up there with him: "Remember that some day the AIDS crisis will be over. And when that day has come and gone there will be people alive on this earth—gay people and straight people, black people and white people, men and women—who will hear the story that once there was a terrible disease, and that a brave group of people stood up and fought and in some cases died so that others might live and be free. I'm proud to be out here today with the people I love, and see the faces of those heroes who are fighting this war, and to be a part of that fight."

There were few there to hear him. And, as I have written, there are few fighting with him. And today the *Times* announced the death of three more friends.

Since I started writing this, I've had a reconciliation with both my brother and sister-in-law. I tried to tell them that I didn't think I'd done anything wrong in writing a blistering letter to one of Arthur's clients for firing a man for his homosexuality. I tried to tell them that I had no other purpose left in my life but fighting for the healthy life of every gay man. They tried to tell me that I didn't understand that my tactics had endangered Arthur's law firm by attacking one of its most important and lucrative clients. I said I found it hard to believe that a letter from Larry would be enough reason for a client to move to another firm after being so ably represented for some dozen years. I said I thought both Arthur and Alice had reacted—it seemed automatically—out of all proportion: sending me letters threatening me that our relationship might be severed, and Arthur writing his client that I was "off the wall" and he would "muzzle" me if he could.

It was after a month of silence that Arthur called and was the first to apologize. We have all those historical reasons for not wanting to rupture our ties. Our mother has drummed into us from the beginning that we must love each other. And we do. Yes, he finally called, as he always does, after my long silence. I sometimes think it's easier for him to apologize than to talk about the issue.

We've had a couple of lunches since he called. The first was strained, he trying to move on and I insisting on my pound of flesh. The second lunch was better. Governor Dukakis had made his acceptance speech and he'd mentioned the word "AIDS." He'd done even more than that. He'd actually said to all the world, "I want our young scientists to dedicate their great gifts not to the destruction of life, but to its preservation. . . . I want them to work with us to win the war against AIDS, the greatest public health emergency of our lifetime, and a disease that must be conquered." I told my brother that when I heard Dukakis say that, I found myself sobbing uncontrollably. It was as if some great weight had been lifted from my body. And I realized that if only Ronald Reagan had said these words in June of 1981, I might have many of my five hundred dead friends still alive; I wouldn't have had to spend seven years of my life screaming; I wouldn't have had to write what I am writing now.

Arthur, who has supported Dukakis from the beginning, said, "It was a pretty good speech." I had the *Times* with me, because both he and I were quoted in it that day. (I in an article about ACT UP and he in an article about his law firm. Our mother would be proud.) I read to him from the governor's speech, the part where he quoted John Winthrop, the first governor of Massachusetts, on the idea of community. " 'We must,' said John Winthrop, 'love one another with a pure heart fervently. We must delight in each other, make each other's condition our own, rejoice together, mourn together, and suffer together. We must,' he said, 'be knit together as one, be knit together as one.' " My brother is not as visibly sentimental as I am, but he kissed me when I dropped him at his office after lunch. Then he asked me to please make peace with his wife. And I said I would do no such thing. The ball was in her court.

Alice was a harder person to deal with. She wasn't calling me, and I certainly wasn't going to call her. I'd felt her letter to me to be particularly hateful. I felt I was no longer welcome at her home. I felt I was not wanted at my younger niece Rebecca's high school graduation. I was angry at Alice for even getting involved in something that was between my brother and me. But as his wife, someone instrumental in furthering his career, and in whom he always confided, she thought she had that right, she indicated when we finally had lunch. She didn't accept it as appropriate or comparable when I said that my Rodger, who has been as instrumental in my career and in whom I also confide, didn't take it upon himself to write her a letter, much as he wanted to.

Much to my surprise, it was my older niece, Liza, who had brought this lunch about. I thought it would be my nephew, Andrew, who would be the peacemaker. He's a smart, jolly young man, who has that rare ability to defuse tense situations. (He also gives copies of my novel, *Faggots*, to his gay friends.) Liza is quiet and thoughtful and, like me, has had a difficult time fighting to find out who she is. She'd come into the city for a date and spent the night on my sofa and over breakfast I'd presented my side of the argument. I may have become too melodramatic, but this is what I felt and said: that I had known five hundred men who had died, and that I didn't know why I was still alive, and that I didn't think any of my family had an idea what my life on a daily basis was like, and they should enjoy what little of my life might be left to me, and us, because I might not be around much longer.

Alice called me that same afternoon and we had our lunch. She is a handsome woman, beautiful really. She is tall and slim and dresses exceptionally well. And she is very smart. (She is completing work on her doctorate in Art History.) And, after years of therapy of her own, also quite confrontational. Over the years our relationship has been both good and bad. For all three of us—Arthur and Alice and Larry—my homosexuality has been an issue. Yet even when Alice and I have fought, she's never excluded me from what she always calls "our extended family."

At our lunch (which was before my second lunch with Arthur), I maintained that the subtext of the whole damn mess
between us was not my letter to the corporation but that they
were still ashamed of my homosexuality. She maintained that
this wasn't true, and that they both were proud of me for being
such a fighter, and why did I insist on beating them forever over
the head for how they'd once felt years ago? She was not in an
apologetic mood, and I had determined beforehand that an apol-
ogy was what I was going to get. And I began to think I wasn't
going to get one. And once again to realize that Arthur had
apologized on the phone because that's easier for him than
having a lunch like this. A couple of times I almost got up and
walked out. That's my way of making it easier for myself. Here
is this woman leaning across this small table and staring in-
tensely into my eyes and not budging an inch. For a while it
looked as if I wouldn't have my family anymore. To make my
point, I seem always prepared to take my stand, take it or leave
it, and take my leave. Either you do this or I don't love you
anymore. She seemed to sense this coming and, instead of
avoiding it, she was pounding on like a pile driver. She'd heard
my hyperbolic statements about hating all heterosexuals. Did
that mean I hated her? And Arthur? And Liza and Andy and
Rebecca? She had said she knew my life was enveloped in
death, and she had great sympathy and sadness for me. And
compassion. (A compassion I hadn't shown to the law firm, she
added.) Did I expect them to give up their lives for my cause?
She used the argument that her best friend is dying of cancer
but she didn't expect Alice to spend her life going out to fight
for cancer research. I told her that in all these eight years she
hadn't sent a check to an AIDS organization, nor had she or
Arthur written a letter to all the important people they knew.
Why, Arthur is a big contributor to Dukakis: Had he written to
him about AIDS? She said I'd never asked them to do any of
this. I said why should I have to ask—they should have done
so voluntarily. And months ago Arthur had offered to write to
Dukakis, but then had told me to write the letter and he'd send
it. So why hadn't I written it, she demanded. Because I'm too
busy writing other things, I countered. What could be more
important, she retaliated. I don't want to have to *ask* you to do
anything, I tried again. (Subtext: You should do it without

asking, because you love me, and care.) [Arthur has since written the letter, which closed with: "I would welcome the opportunity to visit with you on the telephone about what role Larry *and I* (italics mine) can play in helping to formulate policy in this area."] We went on and on. I began to realize that Alice was trying to bring the argument to some definite conclusion. She wasn't going to leave this table until she knew something one way or another. I started saying it's not so black and white, it's not so black and white—whether I want to see you again or not. She stared at me and said nothing. Right now I feel estranged, I said, from you, my brother, your kids, your world, and I don't think this is going to go away so quickly, just like that. "Are you saying that you feel nothing for us?" I didn't answer. "Are you saying that you don't have any love for us, or feel our love for you?" She was staring even harder at me across a table in this East Side restaurant where we'd now been talking for so long that all the other customers had long since departed and the staff was now gathered nearby for some sort of lecture from the boss. "Are you saying that all our lives together, and our history, amount to nothing? And that you don't care for us or love us?" "No, I'm not saying that," I said softly. And she started to cry. And I leaned across the table and kissed her. And I started to cry, too.

Afterword

S ince I completed this book, George Bush has been elected President.

The Presidential Commission's Report on the HIV Epidemic has become the forgotten document many predicted it would become.

Neither Michael Dukakis, nor anyone on his staff, responded to the letter my brother, Arthur, wrote to him about AIDS.

The Institute for Immunological Disorders in Houston, this country's first AIDS hospital, has long since closed its doors for lack of local or national support.

The New York Times has promoted its chief AIDS reporter, Philip Boffey, to the position of Deputy Science Editor.

When asked during one of the Presidential debates to elect a "hero," George Bush named Dr. Anthony Fauci.

Dr. Vincent Devita has left his stewardship of the National Cancer Institute to become one of the heads of Sloan-Kettering, at a reported salary in excess of $400,000 a year.

Just Say No, my political farce about the Reagan-Koch years, was produced. Its theme is that the true root cause for AIDS being ignored is the sexual hypocrisies of our "leaders."

The New York Times critic said, "Imagine the worst possible taste, then take it several steps further."

Ed Koch is running for an unprecedented fourth term.

George Bush's position on AIDS and other gay-related issues is either unknown or frightening.

Not one of the long list of promising drugs and treatments mentioned throughout this book has yet received adequate study or attention at the NIH or FDA.

83,231 and counting . . .

Afterword to the
Paperback Edition

Many things have actually, finally, happened.

The hopeful news is that a number of treatments are emerging that may well turn AIDS into a manageable illness, and that—largely due to the negotiating powers of ACT UP and Project Inform—these treatments will be available years earlier than formerly possible under inhumane "business as usual" FDA regulations.

Indeed, in the past six months ACT UP has wrought a revolution that will change the drug bureaucracy forever. In the past six months, ACT UP has been able to accomplish more than all the gay and AIDS organizations put together have been able to accomplish in the almost ten years of this epidemic. Together with Martin Delaney of San Francisco's Project Inform, ACT UP has presided over the beginning of the breakup of the FDA's brutal control over what we are permitted to do in an attempt to save our own lives.

ACT UP has finally figured the system out. It hasn't been easy. The system doesn't like to be figured out by outsiders. Washington is a byzantine place, filled with swamps, labyrinths, shifting sands, tar pits, and mirages. Just when you think you've found the right person to call, the power shifts to another number, in another building, in another part of town. But ACT UP has pinned the faceless, no-necked monsters to the mat: starting with dogged, continuing, perpetual demonstrations at every possible point of opposition—the FDA, the NIH, HHS, AIDS conferences, and meetings of every description and all over the world; following this with the identification of promising treatments, requesting meetings with their manufacturers, threatening boycotts and demonstrations if refused, and then negotiating with them for the earliest compassionate release of these products; wrapping all this activity in intense media coverage; and capping all this by writing the government's position papers of what must be accomplished, both immediately and in the long run, presenting these documents to the bureaucrats in charge, widely circulating them to all and sundry and then shepherding these position papers into presentation at the relevant conferences and meetings, and demanding and obtaining seats on the new committees formed to approve the release of the very drugs ACT UP negotiated for with their manufacturers in the first place. Yes, ACT UP has succeeded in forcing the system to finally let the people AIDS is happening to have a major voice in what is being done to us.

How has ACT UP accomplished all of this, and in so short a time? Basically by educating ourselves so well that we have answers before anyone else does. Under the leadership of Dr. Iris Long, ACT UP's Treatment + Data Committee has learned more than most scientists and doctors: how drugs work (and don't work), how the FDA works (and doesn't work), how the protocols set up by the National Institute of Allergy and Infectious Diseases work (and don't work). It's taken two years to educate thoroughly and completely, to create these experts. Jim Eigo, Mark Harrington (two brilliant young men who both devote their entire lives to ACT UP), Ken Wylie, David Kirschenbaum, Richard Elovich, Bob Huff, Gary Kleinman, Rebecca Smith, backed up by a sharp team of some thirty other men and women are now so smart that the folks in Washington call *them*. A superb media committee, headed by Jay Blotcher, always in tandem with ACT UP's original fuel—taking to the streets—makes all this operate on a continuing basis. "You guys have all the clout now," an executive at Schering Plough said to me last week, the same pharmaceutical manufacturer which had refused to meet with us for over a year but which has now called and agreed to a meeting. It's almost too good to be true.

Through ACT UP's leadership, the previous inability of the AIDS community to network and cooperate is also slowly changing. A new consensus is emerging that includes Project Inform (led by the great hero, the now grand old man of treatment advocacy, Martin Delaney), AmFar, Lambda Legal Defense, the Community Research Initiative, and ACT UP chapters in other cities, particularly San Francisco, Boston, Chicago, and Los Angeles. Sadly, only Gay Men's Health Crisis has, once again, failed to recognize that a corner has been turned, and also failed to join in truly genuine cooperation. But with them or without them, the grass roots movement of advocacy led by ACT UPs everywhere is paying off.

Yes, miracle of miracle, the government is slowly beginning to respond. It is even possible, or so rumor has it, (God forbid they should be *seen* to be doing anything), George Bush's White House might actually want the AIDS epidemic to end and are gently passing these new words around—in so doing at last breaking the genocidal hex of eight years of Reagan's trickle-down words of do-nothingness. Bush's Secretary of Health and Human Services, Dr. Louis Sullivan, so far seems little more than useless, but in Dr. James Mason, the new Assistant Secretary, we appear to have a man of action, who wants things done, and done quickly. He has also shown great personal compassion toward the epidemic, taking a particular interest in the National Association of People with AIDS.

I would like to convey a special note of thanks to someone whom I criticized most severely in these pages, Dr. Anthony Fauci. In crusading for the notion of "parallel track"—a plan for making experimental drugs available while they are still in

Phase Two efficacy protocols under the FDA, in so doing bringing them to us a minimum of two years faster—he has indeed become the "hero" George Bush once named him. I now salute him, as must we all. It takes great courage for someone to alter so radically his position, admit he's wrong, and so energetically (and radically—Tony now sounds like a member of ACT UP) start out on a new path—a path that is also inherently critical of the work of his fellow bureaucrats.

That this good news is finally present is mostly because of the bad news. There is, as I write this, one new AIDS death every half hour, and there are 212 new AIDS cases every day and one new HIV infection every minute. There will be 100,000 new cases of AIDS in the next fifteen months. (The first 100,000 took nine years). The government has no choice but finally to acknowledge that everything is as awful as we predicted it would be, that everything is out of control, and that the government doesn't quite know what to do. It's almost as if they're saying: might as well listen to the dying faggots—they might even have a few ideas—they couldn't come up with anything worse—anyway, we have to be seen to be trying to do *something*.

With this attitude, we must use every second, every single moment, to press our advantage. The door has been opened and we must get as many feet, fingers, legs, arms, and tongues through it as we can. It could very easily slam in our faces at any minute. ACT UP is riding high now, but some Jesse Helms could come along and find legislative ways to try and silence us.

If we have turned a corner and entered an Age of Treatment, and in so doing entered as well an Age of Hope, there are a few important things not to forget. These drugs we're fighting to get hold of faster might not work for very long. AZT is not a cure but a life-extender. What's in the pipeline to take its place? Are the other drugs ACT UP is fighting for just going to be further extenders, and for how long? And what happens where there aren't any more extenders? And is the early release of anything motivated by a government that just wants to get us off their backs?

So there's no time for celebration or complacency. Everything ahead of us still requires a fight of one sort or another. Research still must be fought for furiously. Accessibility to official treatment protocols still must be fought for. Insurance—more than ever—must be fought for. And *all* AIDS and gay organizations in Washington and elsewhere are going to have to get off their butts and pitch in.

The bad news is that Ed Koch and Mario Cuomo and Daniel Patrick Moynihan and George Bush and politicians everywhere still lie through their teeth publicly about almost everything concerning AIDS and how their cities and states and this country is coping and what the figures are and what the estimates reveal and how totally unprepared we still are. And they are still aided and abetted by generally mediocre media coverage everywhere. *The New York Times*, which somehow still operates under the delusion that it presents "all the news that's fit to print" manages—despite continued ACT UP protests—to be woefully insensitive and inaccurate. There may be more stories, but they're not journalism's pride.

And there is still little good that can yet be said about that supreme horror show which is the Food and Drug Administration. The more I come to fathom the entire drug delivery system in this country, the more I come to see that more people die on a regular basis because they *can't* get unapproved drugs than would ever die from receiving them—that the elaborate machinery our government has thrown up to protect us from the "unsafe" actually does the reverse. America has been in the Stone Age in this whole area; we must study Sweden, Germany, Italy, Britain, Japan, France—where regulations are much less stringent, where drugs come to market with much greater speed, and where consequently people don't seem to be dying in droves.

People who maintain they only want "safe" drugs don't seem to realize that people die on "safe" drugs, too. All those who want drugs without any side effects don't seem to realize there's probably never going to be any such thing, or if there is it will be too weak to work. People forget that approved forms of chemotherapy have many side effects, and kill many people, or don't work on many people; but they also work on many people, too. And AZT (or ddI or DDC or GM-CSF) is chemotherapy.

On a personal note, I've tested HIV-positive, as I suspected I would. (Yes, I think The Test—if you have insurance and access to adequate health care, and at least 35 million Americans don't—is ready to be taken now, because treatments are available that have been proved to prolong life.) No amount of that suspicion matches the actuality of discovering the truth. Even though there is nothing different in my body except this new bit of information in my mind, my life is changed forever. A new fear has now joined my daily repertoire of emotions, and my nighttime ones, too. But life has also become exceptionally more precious and, ironically, I am happier. And because of my involvement with ACT UP, I feel productive and well-used.

ACT UP gives me my greatest energy, and my greatest commitment to staying alive. Each week I go to meetings, tired at the end of a long day, and emerge euphoric. I now know more than ever the empowerment that comes from activism. I feel satisfaction in realizing that what I've written about endlessly for so many years can actually work in practice. We have been rude and we have been smart and we have been united and it works. Yes, this makes me feel good. Had I only been able to stay at GMHC and work toward this same revolution nine years earlier! But it is the new, young generation that is ACT UP. GMHC was founded by the older and the more polite. I hate politeness.

Surely ACT UP has taught everyone that you don't get anything by being nice, good little boys and girls. You do not get more with honey than with vinegar. Oh, how I've said this all along. Oh, how I was maligned and screamed at and condemned and made into a pariah. I'm often asked if it feels good to have been proved right. I usually duck the question; there's always so much more that has yet to be done to ever sit still complacently for a second. Now that I must face the harshest of all realities, my own mortality, I'm trying to be less hard on myself. I try to take a smidgin of satisfaction knowing that the two main AIDS organizations in this world are there because they were my idea. But the minute I even allow myself to think such thoughts, I remember dead friends and lovers and acquaintances who might still be here had everyone—myself included—fought a little bit harder. And I realize that I'm robbed of comfort by the fury I never seem to get over against my gay and straight do-nothing friends and all the gay and AIDS organizations filled with nice, good little boys and girls.

How can we turn millions of nice, good little boys and girls into warriors filled with vinegar? The war isn't over and there is no army that doesn't need all the fighters it can get. The battle is now for speed, for hurry, to make tomorrow happen today. One new HIV infection every minute. One new AIDS death every half hour. Two hundred and twelve new AIDS cases every day. There are many of us yet to die. Unless . . . Unless . . .

Mark Harrington, who studied these things at Harvard, is fond of saying that the world's revolutions did not happen when there was no hope. They happen when there *is* hope, and when the system can't keep up with the rising expectations of the maligned and downtrodden. With AZT and aerosolized pentamadine and Bactrim and ddI, and after that who knows how many miraculous-sounding things, we have hope. I once worried that one Monday night I'd walk into an ACT UP meeting and no one would be there. The movement would have fizzled out. But each week there are *more* people there. And each month there is a new chapter formed in another town or city. The revolution *has* started.

Yes, there is certainly something abroad in the land that was not around when I completed *Reports from the holocaust*. It's called hope, and I, for one, plan—one of these days—to glory in it.

105,990 and counting . . .

September 1989